INSTITUTE OF PSYCHIATRY

Maudsley Monographs

MARRIAGE AND FERTILITY OF WOMEN SUFFERING FROM SCHIZOPHRENIA OR AFFECTIVE DISORDERS

INSTITUTE OF PSYCHIATRY

MAUDSLEY MONOGRAPHS

Number Nineteen

MARRIAGE AND FERTILITY OF WOMEN SUFFERING FROM SCHIZOPHRENIA OR AFFECTIVE DISORDERS

By

BARBARA C. STEVENS

B.A., Ph.D.

Member of the Scientific Staff, Medical Research Council Social Psychiatry Research Unit, Institute of Psychiatry, The Maudsley Hospital, London

Previous Holder of the Mapother Fellowship, Medical Research Council

LONDON

OXFORD UNIVERSITY PRESS

NEW YORK   TORONTO

1969

Oxford University Press, London W.1

GLASGOW NEW YORK TORONTO MELBOURNE WELLINGTON
CAPE TOWN SALISBURY IBADAN NAIROBI LUSAKA ADDIS ABABA
BOMBAY CALCUTTA MADRAS KARACHI LAHORE DACCA
KUALA LUMPUR SINGAPORE HONG KONG TOKYO

PRINTED IN GREAT BRITAIN BY
THE CAMELOT PRESS LTD, LONDON AND SOUTHAMPTON

CONTENTS

Preface   vii

Acknowledgements   ix

PART 1. REVIEW OF THE LITERATURE

   I. Historical Introduction   I
  II. Systematic Empirical Investigations   5
 III. Genetic and Social Relevance of the Problem   22

PART 2. AIMS AND PILOT INQUIRIES

  IV. Statement of the Problem, and Pilot Inquiries on Methods of
      Sample Selection   33
   V. The Aims of the Main Inquiry on Women of Childbearing
      Age   38

PART 3. METHODOLOGY OF THE MAIN INQUIRY

  VI. Methods of Sample Selection in the Main Inquiry   43
 VII. Methods of Collecting Data   47
VIII. Statistical Methods and Data Processing   60

PART 4. RESULTS

   IX. Clinical and Social Structure of the Sample   67
    X. Probability of Marriage Before First Admission   76
  XI. Probability of Marriage After First Admission   85
 XII. Legitimate Fertility Before First Admission   97
XIII. Legitimate Fertility After First Admission   105
XIV. Changes in Marital Status: Separation and Divorce   119
 XV. Illegitimate Fertility   132
XVI. Miscellaneous Data   139
XVII. Reliability of Data   148

PART 5. DISCUSSION AND CONCLUSIONS

XVIII. Discussion of Results in Relation to Those of Previous Studies   159
 XIX. Conclusions   169

      References   171

      Index   179

MAUDSLEY MONOGRAPHS

HENRY MAUDSLEY, from whom this series of monographs takes its name, was the founder of The Maudsley Hospital and the most prominent English psychiatrist of his generation. The Maudsley Hospital is now united with Bethlem Royal Hospital. and its medical school, renamed the Institute of Psychiatry, has become part of the British Postgraduate Medical Federation. It is entrusted by the University of London with the duty to advance psychiatry by teaching and research.

The monograph series reports work carried out in the Institute and in the associated Hospital. Some of the monographs are directly concerned with clinical problems; others, less obviously relevant, are in scientific fields that are cultivated for the furtherance of psychiatry.

Joint Editors

PROFESSOR SIR DENIS HILL
F.R.C.P., D.P.M.

PROFESSOR J. T. EAYRS
Ph.D., D.SC.

PREFACE

THIS book describes the first survey in England to estimate the probability of marriage and fertility of women suffering from schizophrenia and affective disorders since the development of community-orientated psychiatry.

Over 1,300 women suffering from these disorders were selected from admissions to a London psychiatric hospital during the years 1955–63, and they were followed up after discharge until August 1966. The gradual movement away from certification and custodial care of psychotics towards day- and out-patient care, and routine supervision of medication by general practitioners had profoundly influenced the family lives of these patients. Probability of marriage of these patients, before and after admission, was compared with that of normal women of corresponding age observed during identical calendar periods, as derived from the Registrar General's Statistical Estimates for England and Wales. The analysis of fertility controlled for age at marriage and duration of marriage in comparison with general population data, and the study of the period after admission was designed especially to measure the role of hospitalization in reducing exposure to conception. An attempt was made to assess the frequency of separation and divorce of these patients and their illegitimate fertility in comparison with indices derived from published data on women in the general population.

The results indicated a lessening of differentials between patients and normal women since the development of community care. However, the finding of particular clinical and social importance was that before illness the probability of marriage of schizophrenic women was only three-quarters of the probability of corresponding women and after illness the probability of marriage of schizophrenic women was further reduced to just over one-third of normal. The legitimate fertility of the schizophrenics was reduced both before and after illness to a statistically significant extent, but much of the latter reduction depended on the role of hospitalization, and the differentials were too small to be of any real eugenic importance. Probability of marriage and fertility of women suffering from affective disorders was very similar to that of the corresponding general population of women.

This research is an example of the application of modern demographic analysis to psychiatric problems, and the results cannot be fully understood without reference to the methodology involved. The author would like to suggest the following plan of reading for those whose time is limited: CHAPTERS V to VIII on aims and methods are essential, and then there is a brief summary of the main findings at the end of each chapter in the Results

Section. The DISCUSSION and CONCLUSIONS have been kept as short as possible to permit a concise presentation of the clinical and sociological significance of the survey.

London   B. S.
1969

ACKNOWLEDGEMENTS

I SHOULD like to thank Mr. N. H. Carrier, Reader in Demography at the London School of Economics for his enormous help in the design and mathematical analysis of this study and for his never failing kindness and support. Thanks are particularly due to Professor Sir Aubrey Lewis, who suggested this subject for investigation, for his excellent supervision and encouragement, and whose example of academic learning has always been an inspiration to me. I am especially grateful to Professor David Glass, who initially encouraged my interest in social psychiatry, for his supervision and expert advice, to Miss Susannah Brown for her mathematical advice, to Dr. J. K. Wing for assessing the reliability of diagnosis, and to Professor Sir Denis Hill and Miss Hague for their careful advice on the preparation of the manuscript.

The research was made possible by the award of the Mapother Fellowship of the Medical Research Council, for which I am very grateful. Thanks are especially due to Dr. H. C. Beccle and Dr. M. Markowe for excellent facilities provided at their hospital, to my research assistants especially Mr. Daniel Appadou and Mr. Nigel Kalton, and to Mr. P. Wakeford for permitting the use of his Social Survey Computer Programme at the London School of Economics. I am particularly indebted to Miss Christine Durston for reliable and skilful secretarial help.

I should like to thank all those hospitals and general practitioners who co-operated in the follow-up inquiry, and all the Borough Councils and N.H.S. Executive Councils which helped me to trace patients. I am especially grateful to Dr. B. Benjamin and Mr. Rooke Matthews of the General Register Office for their help in tracing patients via the N.H.S. Central Register. I am also especially grateful for all the help given to me by the patients, upon whose lives this research is based.

Part 1. Review of the Literature

CHAPTER I

HISTORICAL INTRODUCTION

DURING the nineteenth century, interest in the fertility of psychiatric patients was stimulated by two main historical trends; first the development of statistics and their application to problems of human populations, and secondly, the impact of Darwinian theories and the resultant concern over concepts of degeneracy.

1. Early Interest in Demographic Aspects of Psychiatry

In France, Philippe Pinel was perhaps the first psychiatrist to write on the application of statistical theory to problems concerning patients in hospital (1806). He wrote articles on the ratio of male to female births, and on the need for follow-up studies on methods of psychiatric treatment, but the fertility of his patients did not seem to interest him.

In England, William Farr seems to have been the first medical statistician to write an official report on the mentally ill (1835). In *Statistics of English Lunatic Asylums and the Reform of their Public Management* he gave details of admissions, deaths, and finance for hospitals throughout England and Wales. Farr claimed that pauper lunatics and idiots made up 0·00098 or one in 1,024 of the total population, and he gave an estimate of patients in public and private asylums and those in the care of Parish Officers.

After Farr, Thurnam in York wrote a paper, published in the *American Journal of Insanity* in 1845, on the relative liability of the two sexes to insanity. He analysed admissions to asylums in Europe and America, taking into account the proportion of men and women exposed in the general population and concluded that men were more liable than women to insanity. A growing body of statistics developed during the nineteenth century which paved the way to the early empirical work on the fertility of psychiatric patients. Some writers, as early as 1849, were distrustful of figures and Baillarger (1849) claimed, for example, in writing to Renaudin that 'The evil is in the disconnection and want of similarity of methods of investigation', and emphasized that there must be large samples for statistics to be truly valuable and that they should be based on a common conceptual framework. Towards the end of the century, articles in the *Journal of Mental Science* showed the growing concern about the outcome of different classes of insanity; for example, Tuke (1880) attempted to tabulate recoveries, and Chapman (1880) attempted to analyse the mortality of patients in four asylums in England and Wales, taking into consideration diagnosis, age, sex, and length of stay.

The nineteenth-century statistics of insanity were concentrated on the problems of liability and curability and mortality of the mentally ill. In an age when poverty, custodial care and high mortality were the concern of psychiatrists, it is hardly surprising that the question of fertility is not raised. It was not until the impact of Darwinism awakened interest in the inheritance of insanity that the first empirical work on fertility was begun.

Theories of Degeneracy

The concept of degenerate types can be traced to Sylvius (1556), but not until the nineteenth century was the concept applied to the study of psychiatric patients (see Walter, 1956, on the history of the concept of degeneracy).

In France, Morel (1857) considered that degeneration was the moral depravities of the parents being transmitted to the offspring; the first generation would thus contain a high proportion of neurotics, criminals, and paupers, the second generation would involve more insane and mental defectives until finally defects would be so severe as to produce sterility of the tainted family. Maudsley (1862), perhaps influenced by Morel, wrote 'Insanity of what form soever, whether mania, melancholia, moral insanity, or dementia, is but a step in the descent toward sterile idiocy' but he did not carry out any systematic statistical work on the fertility of his patients.

Adolf Meyer in America was the first psychiatrist to offer a more constructive approach to the problem, and following, perhaps unwittingly, the ideas of Farr, recommended the registration of the insane, and went further than Farr, in suggesting a study of the intermarriage of patients (1895). Meyer quotes Luys (1895) on 'Reciprocal morbid attraction of the insane', in which fourteen patients who married each other were sterile or produced degenerate offspring.

Evolutionary theories stimulated further interest in the fertility of psychiatric patients and in the early twentieth century eugenists considered that this might be in excess of that found in the general population. Leonard Darwin (1926) claimed that 'defective intelligence is undoubtedly associated with great fertility, it is not therefore surprising to learn that thieves and other petty offenders spring from amongst the most fertile stocks in the community'. Further confusion of moral ideas with problems of scientific fact can be found in Armstrong's *The Survival of the Unfittest* (1927) and even, to a lesser extent, in general medicine in Pende's *Constitutional Inadequacies* (1928).

A controversy arose regarding the sterility or excessive fertility of psychiatric patients, and as Lewis (1958) demonstrates the early empirical work of the Eugenics Laboratory in London may only be fully understood with reference to the above concepts, which were prevalent at the time.

Early Empirical Studies on the Fertility of Psychotics

The first statistical inquiry into the fertility of psychiatric patients was by Heron (1907) under the auspices of the Francis Galton Eugenics Laboratory. Heron obtained a sample of 331 families, one member of each being in Perth Asylum in Scotland. He grouped all the mentally-ill patients together, because of diagnostic differences which experts could not agree upon, and he quotes Dr. Sankey in support of this: 'Insanity is but the process, and the so-called varieties are merely differentiated by non-essential phenomena, that all insanities begin with melancholia, and tend to pass through a succession of stages in the order—melancholia, mania, dementia—a succession liable at any time to interruption by recovery.'

Heron calculated the number of sibships of each size, one member of each being mentally ill, and obtained a mean family size of 5·97; he also had a group of eighty-seven fertile marriages in which one parent was insane, and obtained a mean family size of 5·18. In comparing this with Pearson's mean of 6·6 for English fertile marriages of fifteen years' duration, and Westergaard's mean of 5·18 for Danish professional classes of the same duration, Heron concluded that the insane must be at least as fertile or more fertile than the general population of a similar social class and length of marriage. Heron indicated that no reduction in fertility was found, in spite of the fact that some of his patients had been confined in the asylum for long periods since marriage. Although he wrote on the need for large unbiassed samples and the importance of controlling for social variables, neither of these methodological criteria was achieved by his sample; he did not take into account age at and duration of marriage adequately, nor social class, in his comparisons with Pearson's and Westergaard's work on samples from the general population.

However, Pearson (1909) agreed with Heron's conclusion, and in confusing the statistical problems with moral issues, he claimed that the humanitarian care of degenerate types was preventing the survival of the fittest; Pearson quotes Plato (*Laws V*) as the first eugenist to advocate that degenerates be deported and that 'the intellectual oligarchy should aim at social purification'.

The factual basis for these authoritarian views was criticized by Weinberg (1910 and 1913) and finally by Greenwood and Yule (1914) in a paper 'On the determination of the size of the family, and of the distribution of characters in order of birth from samples taken through members of sibships'. They showed the eugenists that Heron's claim that the fertility of abnormal groups was in excess of the normal was statistically invalid, in that he over-estimated the true mean by 25–50 per cent by incurring a bias towards large families: smaller sibships were less likely to contain a mentally-ill member and were therefore less likely to be selected. Greenwood and Yule corrected Heron's mean family size of psychiatric patients to between 4·06 and 4·38, and further criticized Heron's use of χ^2 on such a small sample where the normal distribution may not apply. Edgeworth (1914), then President of the Royal Statistical

Society, finally concluded in the discussion of Greenwood and Yule's paper that the earlier work on the fertility of the mentally ill was based on statistical fallacies, involving the application of inappropriate mathematical statistics to small samples.

In view of these criticisms it is surprising that no further systematic inquiries on the fertility of the mentally ill appeared in this country until after the Second World War.

In the following review of the literature, and throughout this monograph, the meaning of the term fertility is essentially demographic, and refers to the number of children actually born alive to a woman; the average number of children born to a specific group of married women is often called the mean family size of the group. This concept of fertility should not be confused with the medical meaning of the term referring to fecundity, or the biological capacity of a woman to bear a child, which was implied by early writers such as Maudsley in their confusion of moral issues with problems of scientific fact. The controlled demographic studies of the fertility of the mentally ill were first undertaken by German and American investigators.

CHAPTER II

SYSTEMATIC EMPIRICAL INVESTIGATIONS

TABLE I summarizes fifteen previous studies on the marriage and fertility of psychiatric patients; seven of these were on German or Scandinavian samples, four were based on American patients, and two were on patients admitted to hospitals serving the London area.

Previous research has failed to achieve the necessary methodological sophistication needed to estimate, in an unbiased manner, the total fertility of schizophrenics compared with manic depressives. Large representative samples are necessary, and in order to compare these patients with corresponding groups in the general population, there must be adequate control of variables known to influence the probability of marrying, and fertility, in modern societies. The effect of these illnesses on fertility may only be analysed by such careful and controlled comparisons, and the results of previous research which omitted such methodology should be considered unreliable. The literature may be reviewed in terms of the extent to which it has contributed to our knowledge of *total fertility* of psychiatric patients: the main components of this being the proportion married, and fertility before and after first admission.

Studies on Proportions Married on First Psychiatric Admission

Myerson (1917), Dayton (1940), Brugger (1931), and Norris (1956) have all given estimates of proportions of patients ever married on admission to mental hospitals. However, they did not relate this to marriage rates after discharge or to fertility.

Myerson took all admissions to Taunton State Hospital, U.S.A., for the period 1854–1916, and obtained 500 cases of each sex diagnosed as suffering from dementia praecox. He found lowered proportions ever married for both sexes compared with those in the general population of a similar age. For example, out of 309 males aged 20–34 years on admission 18 per cent were ever married, compared with 49 per cent in the general population; in his group of women the reduction was also apparent, but to a lesser extent. Myerson concluded that there is an inborn tendency in schizophrenics against self-perpetuation, especially in the male; he did not quote his source of data on the general population but it seems likely that the age structure of his patients aged 20–34 was biassed towards the younger ages and therefore not strictly comparable with the general population of this group. We cannot, therefore, fully accept his results.

Dayton (1940) analysed over 89,000 admissions to Massachusetts State mental hospitals during the years 1917–33 and showed, as Myerson had done, the

TABLE 1

SUMMARY OF PREVIOUS STUDIES ON MARRIAGE AND FERTILITY OF SCHIZOPHRENICS AND MANIC-DEPRESSIVES

(In chronological order of samples)

Author	Sample	Results on marriage	Results on fertility
Heron (1907)	331 families, 1 member of each being in Perth Asylum, Scotland	Not studied	Mean family size = 5·97 higher than general population. Corrected to 3·34 by Popenoe (less than general population)
Myerson (1917)	500 schizophrenic men and 500 schizophrenic women admitted to Taunton Hospital, U.S.A., 1854–1916	Lowered proportion ever married	Not studied
Kallmann (1938)	Schizophrenics (1,087) admitted to Berlin Hospital, 1893–1902. Followed-up until 1930s	Lowered proportion ever married before and after admission in all groups except paranoids	Reduced fertility before and after admission, especially in catatonic and simplex cases
Dahlberg (1933)	2,200 admissions (all diagnoses) to Swedish Hospitals, 1890–1929	Lowered proportion married in all groups of patients	Reduced legitimate and illegitimate fertility
Popenoe (1928 a and b)	All U.S.A. admissions 1922 (Popenoe 1928a). Sample of sterilized and non-sterilized patients in California (Popenoe 1928b)	Lowered proportion ever married schizophrenics and manic-depressives	Mean family size = 2·16 (sterilized female schizophrenics) and 1·63 (non-sterilized schizophrenics)
Essen-Möller (1935)	Over 4,000 admissions 1904–27 to Munich Psychiatric Clinic, schizophrenics and manic-depressives followed up till 1931	Lowered probability of marriage before and more so after illness in schizophrenics. Manic-depressives only differ from normals after illness	Fertility of schizophrenic women is reduced but schizophrenic men lagged behind general decline in birth rate. Manic-depressives only differ after discharge
Böök (1953)	Entire incidence 1902–49, North Swedish isolate	Lowered probability of marriage in schizophrenics	High legitimate fertility of schizophrenics compared with normal controls
Dayton (1940)	All admissions to Massachusetts hospitals, U.S.A., 1917–33	Lowered proportion married on admission in all groups	Not studied
Brugger (1931)	73 schizophrenics from Census of patients in Thuringia, 1931	Lowered proportion ever married	Not studied
Nissen (1932)	Scandinavian small sample, schizophrenics 1932	Lowered proportion ever married	Reduced fertility
Ødegaard (1960)	1936–55 admissions Norway, and small follow-up of 817 cases	Lowered proportion married in schizophrenics	High legitimate fertility of schizophrenics compared with manic-depressives
Norris (1956)	8,000 admissions (all diagnoses) to London mental hospitals	Single patients are over-represented on admission and stay in hospital longer	Not studied
Erlenmeyer-Kimling, Rainer, and Kallmann (1966)	Over 1,600 admissions of schizophrenics 1934–6, 1954–6 New York. Followed-up until 1961	Increased proportion single in schizophrenics before illness but recent series demonstrate an increased proportion married	A lessening of fertility differentials in recent series
M. Fakhr El-Islam and Hend A. El-Deeb (1968)	67 male and 65 female schizophrenics, 40 male and 68 female manic-depressives attending an Arab out-patient clinic in 1966 compared with a matched control sample of general medical out-patients	Excess of single patients among the schizophrenics, especially those of schizoid personality	Reduced fertility of schizophrenics
Shearer, Cain, Finch, and Davidson (1968)	Comparative study of the fertility rates of in-patients in Michigan Hospitals, 1935–64	Not studied	Increase of 366 per cent in the fertility rate *within* the hospitals, comparing the rate of 1935–9 with the rate for 1960–4, i.e. increase since an 'open door' policy

excess of single patients in all diagnostic groups. However, Dayton did not try to analyse proportions marrying by diagnoses, although he related sociological variables to marital status categories. Taking all diagnoses together, he compared the proportion married among patients from urban and rural environments with that found in the 1920 Census reports, and discovered that the married were still under-represented. His comparisons did not allow for yearly variations in the marriage rate, but they do indicate the tendency for *all* psychiatric patients towards low marriage rates. This suggests that there may be an inherent bias towards the single in samples based on mental hospital admissions—a bias not necessarily due to schizophrenia or determinants associated with schizoid personality, but resulting from the fact that single people have no one to look after them and are more in need of beds, or some such sociological rather than clinical explanation.

Brugger (1931) took a census of psychiatric patients in Thuringia, Germany, and found a lowered proportion married among the schizophrenics. His sample was, however, far too small (under 100) for reliable conclusions. Norris (1956) analysed 8,000 admissions to London mental hospitals and showed that single schizophrenic patients are over-represented on admission, especially among the men. Norris also indicated that single patients were more likely to stay in hospital longer than married patients. Norris gave no clear estimation of proportions ever married on first admission by diagnosis compared with the general population of London, and therefore it appears that no basic index of marriage before illness can be derived from her data.

The above studies suggest that schizophrenics may exhibit a lowered marriage rate before they become ill, and that this may be especially important in the male schizophrenic group. But lack of adequate control data makes it impossible to obtain precise estimates from these studies.

Studies of Marriage and Fertility BEFORE First Psychiatric Admission

Popenoe (1928 a and b), Nissen (1932), Dahlberg (1933), and MacSorley (1964) have all attempted to study proportions married and legitimate fertility before first psychiatric admission.

Popenoe's aim was to discover the eugenic value of sterilization in California, rather than to obtain an unbiassed estimate of fertility of his patients. However, he gave data on marriage for all first admissions to United States mental hospitals in 1922: 59 per cent of schizophrenic women and 75 per cent of manic-depressive women were ever married compared with 88 per cent in the general population of California, aged 34–44 in the 1920 Census. The corresponding proportions for men were 28 per cent for schizophrenics and 59 per cent for manic-depressives. Popenoe did not correct for the differential age at marriage between them. Thus his findings tend to agree with Myerson, Brugger, and Norris on the lowered proportions ever married of schizophrenics before their first admission, particularly in the case of male schizophrenics.

Popenoe (1928a) made a further contribution in this field when he attempted to discover why this low marriage rate existed. Mott (1919) and Gibbs (1924–5) claimed that cases of dementia praecox exhibited a lack of normal hetero-sexual drive, the basis of which may be endocrinological. Mott's histological studies suggested the existence of testicle atrophy in male schizophrenics. Gibbs found that a masculine distribution of pubic hair occurred four to five times more frequently in female dementia praecox cases than in a control group of mixed diagnoses and this seemed to be related to sexual immaturity and, in some cases, to overt homosexuality. Popenoe investigated a small sample of schizophrenics and found they had as much heterosexual experience as a control group of other diagnoses; he drew no conclusions regarding the reason for the low marriage rate of schizophrenics before illness, nor could he discover any evidence to suggest that men or women of more positive heredity of insanity were discriminated against in marriage selection; although this factor seemed more important in women than in men.

Popenoe (1928b) also studied the fertility of sterilized patients compared with that of a control sample of patients who had not been sterilized; all the sterilized groups demonstrated a higher mean family size than the controls; for example, 250 married sterilized women suffering from dementia praecox had a mean family size of 2·16 compared with the mean of 1·63 of the 48 women of the control group of this diagnosis. The group of over 400 manic-depressives, who had been sterilized, had a mean family size of 2·29 compared with that of 1·50 of 40 controls who had not been sterilized. These differences were not statistically significant. However, Popenoe noted that 15 per cent of the married sterilized group (all diagnoses) were childless, compared with 33 per cent of the married controls. Considering estimates, and taking the low proportions married into account, he concluded that the mentally ill in California were not replacing themselves, indeed only about half of them would ever bear children.

Popenoe corrected Heron's mean family size for all psychotics to 3·34 by a formula similar to that proposed by Greenwood and Yule (1914) and sugges-ted that any increase in the numbers of insane was not due to the fertility of their parents, but came from patients whose parents were not insane, but who carried the recessive genes for insanity. Popenoe attempted no demographic analysis by age at and duration of marriage, nor by social class, and he did not publish comparative data from the general population on fertility.

Nissen (1932) published further evidence, based on a Scandinavian sample, that schizophrenics exhibit a lowered marriage frequency and fertility when compared with the general population. Nissen's work remains untranslated and therefore cannot be reviewed in detail. Dahlberg (1933) undertook in Sweden an inquiry similar to Dayton's in America on proportions married among 2,200 women admitted to Uppsala Mental Hospital during 1890–1929. He found that for all diagnoses in the age group 45 and over, 55 per cent of his patients were ever married, compared with 81 per cent in the corresponding general population. These results agree with those of Dayton's on all patients, and with Myerson's, Norris', Popenoe's, and Nissen's on schizophrenics. Dahlberg's study gave comparisons with fertility of women in the general population, controlled for age on first admission; the legitimate mean family size of his patients was 3·3, lower than the 3·8 of the general population. Legitimate fertility of patients varied with age on admission from 0·05 for women aged under 20, to 2·5 for women admitted aged over 50. Dahlberg found illegitimate fertility to be very low with a mean of 0·34, and finally concluded that his patients were not replacing themselves. He did not differentiate by diagnoses, and his comparisons with the general population seem uncontrolled for social class, religion and other variables (as reviewed by Lewis, 1958).

One further study has attempted to estimate marriage and fertility before first admission. MacSorley (1964) undertook the sole British investigation since Heron's. Unfortunately her sample was too small for any reliable conclusions to be drawn; she selected 51 schizophrenic men and 48 schizophrenic women, and an even smaller group of paranoid patients admitted to Horton and St. Bernard's Hospitals during 1958–60; only first admissions were selected. She improved on the work of previous workers in selecting a normal control group of about 650 of each sex (who lived in the Hospitals' catchment areas) from the wards of a general hospital, and from two industrial concerns. She also had a small group of 41 male and 58 female depressives. The percentage single in her schizophrenic groups was found to be in excess of that expected on the basis of the controls, and on the basis of estimates derived from the Registrar General's Reviews. The depressives were nearer the percentages expected in the general population.

Taking mean legitimate family size, MacSorley found a mean of 1·6 for non-paranoid schizophrenic women, 1·1 for paranoid cases, and 1·4 for depressives; the corresponding figures for men were 1·6, 1·8, and 1·8 respectively. The controls gave a mean of 2·2 for women and 2·1 for men. She therefore concluded that her patients showed a reduction in their fertility before their first admission, which would agree with the work of previous investigators. She also gave evidence of assortative mating, for example of 117 married female patients, four had psychotic husbands who required treatment. MacSorley did not quote her source of general population data and did not appear to control for age at and duration of marriage, nor for social class, and she made no recommendation regarding the need to study post-psychotic trends in an estimation of total fertility of psychiatric patients.

We may conclude that none of the above studies had provided reliable estimates of the probability of marrying and/or of the fertility of schizophrenics and manic-depressives before their first admission. The work of Myerson, Brugger and MacSorley was based on too small samples, and Dayton's and Dahlberg's large samples failed to discriminate between diagnostic groups. Popenoe was preoccupied with the practical issue of eugenic sterilization, and Norris measured the relation between marital status and the need for hospital care rather than the relation of probability of marriage to fertility.

However, these studies suggest that a lowered probability of marrying and lowered fertility would be expected in schizophrenics before first admission, and this was further discovered by Kallmann and Essen-Möller in their detailed studies of fertility of schizophrenics before and after first admission.

Studies of Fertility of Schizophrenics and Manic-Depressives before and after First Admission with Special Reference to Female Patients

Total fertility of schizophrenics has been estimated by Kallman (1938) in Germany, Böök (1953) in Sweden, and Erlenmeyer-Kimling, Rainer, and Kallmann (1966) in New York. In Munich, Essen-Möller (1935), and in Norway Ødegaard (1960) have attempted to compare the fertility of schizophrenics and manic-depressives. It was decided to study female patients, because data concerning their fertility were easier to obtain from case records, and because the data from the general population in England were more orientated towards fertility of women.

Between 1929 and 1937, Kallmann followed up 1,087 schizophrenic patients admitted before the age of 40 to Herzberg Hospital, Berlin, between 1893 and 1902. He obtained, by intensive interviews with their families, detailed information on marriage, fertility, and incidence of mental and physical disorders for 93·2 per cent of the original sample (although only 23·1 per cent of the patients themselves were alive at the end of the follow-up).

First considering the proportion married, all but the paranoid group of late onset demonstrated a considerably higher proportion single both before and after admission when compared with the general population in Berlin. For example, 40 per cent of the hebephrenic women were ever married on their first psychiatric admission, their mean age at this time being 29·6 years. At the end of the follow-up in 1933 only 42·4 per cent of this group were ever married. In the catatonic group 22·4 per cent married before admission, and only 31·6 per cent were ever married afterwards. However, the simplex group appeared to exhibit a higher rate of marriage after admission: 29·3 per cent were married at this time, with a mean age of 25·2 years compared with 67·4 per cent at the end of observation in 1933. Comparing these indices with the general population, 71 per cent of all adults in Berlin during the years 1890–1900 were ever married. The paranoid women were on average 40·9 years on first admission and from this time 79·6 per cent were ever married, which is probably not significantly different from this age group in the general population. Kallmann estimated that only 30 per cent of all his patients' marriages occurred after first admission, but the high rate among simplex cases during this period demonstrated a need for eugenic counselling. These findings accord with those of previous studies, but Kallmann's comparisons with the general population did not control for variation in age structure, so that it is difficult to assess the reliability of his differentials.

Considering fertility, Kallmann discovered a definite reduction among his non-paranoid schizophrenic probands compared with the fertility of the general population of Germany. Taking a combined index of pre- and post-psychotic births, the hebephrenic probands had a mean family size of 3·5, the catatonics 3·0, and the simplex group 2·1, compared with an estimated mean of between 4·4 and 4·8 for the general population of Germany between the years 1884–1900 (Kallmann, 1938: TABLES 19 and 21, pp. 64 and 66). Paranoid patients whose illness is often of later onset had a comparatively higher mean of 4·6 compared with the others. Kallmann noted that only 38·5 per cent of all fertility occurred after first discharge, and indicated that post-psychotic fertility rates would be increased if the long periods of hospitalization were excluded from the analysis. He attempted to control for socio-economic status in comparing completed fertility of a paranoid-simplex group of late onset with the population of Borken as studied by Muckerman, and concluded that even this group showed a considerably lower proportion of families having four or more children than that found in the general population of Borken. However, most of Kallmann's comparisons failed to control for age at marriage, duration of marriage, religion and social class so that unbiassed estimates of pre- and post-psychotic fertility are difficult to derive from his tabulations.

Essen-Möller (1935) produced more reliable estimates of total fertility of schizophrenics and manic-depressives in Germany during the early part of this century. He selected a total sample of over 4,000 patients suffering from these psychoses from admissions to the Munich Psychiatric Clinic between the years 1904–27; of these patients 1,194 were women with a definite diagnosis of schizophrenia, and 643 women were in the definite depressive category. Unfortunately the sample was not a random one: patients selected from 1904–17 admissions were only those which Rüdin had previously studied, or whose diagnosis had appeared certain; between 1919 and 1927 several hundred admissions were omitted for no clear reason, and 1,000 admissions between 1916 and 1922 were excluded to lessen the work involved, and to contrast the earlier period of admissions before the German birth rate fell, with later admissions when this demographic change was occurring in the general population.

Like Kallmann, Essen-Möller followed up his sample until 1 January 1931, and interviewed the families of 67 per cent of married patients in order to compensate for the fact, discovered in a pilot study, that the official sources of registration of births appeared to underestimate the number of children born. Single patients were only followed up by contacting institutions and official agencies, and therefore this aspect of his follow-up produced a bias towards patients who did not recover. Essen-Möller improved greatly on the work of Kallmann in obtaining a large control sample of 960 marriages registered in Munich during the years 1876–1930 and he also utilized Makela's sample of 279 uncles and aunts of traumatic epileptics in Bavaria, who were shown to be

TABLE 2

FOR SCHIZOPHRENIC WOMEN RECONSTRUCTION OF MARITAL STATUS CATEGORIES BEFORE ILLNESS

Percentage of single women in italics

Length of time from the illness

Age at first admission and entry into the sample →

Age →		15	20	25	30	35	40	45	50	55	60
55	v I	0	0	2	1	1	2	0	0	0	0
	vw, g	0	0	1	0	0	2	0	1	0	0
	Rest	21	21	18	14	14	8	8	7	6	6
	%	*100·0*		*85·7*	*66·7*	*37·7*	*37·7*	*33·3*			*28·6*
50	v I	0	0	2	1	1	1	0	0	0	
	vw, g	0	1	2	1	1	0	0	0	0	
	R	33	32	28	19	19	10	8	8	8	
	%	*100·0*		*84·9*	*57·6*		*30·3*	*24·2*		*24·2*	
45	v 2	0	0	4	5	5	6	2	2	0	
	vw, g	0	0	2	3	3	0	0	0	0	
	R	96	96	86	60	53	41	29	29	8	
	%	*100·0*		*89·6*	*62·5*		*42·7*	*30·2*	*30·2*	*24·2*	
40	v 2	0	0	3	8	8	1	0	0		
	vw, g	1	2	1	1	1	0	0	0		
	R	110	108	101	59	51	48	46	42	42	
	%	*99·1*		*91·0*	*53·2*	*45·9*	*41·4*	*37·*	*37·*		
35	v 2	0	5	5	12	10	12	3			
	vw, g	0	0	2	1	1	0	0			
	R	205	195	183	124	104	80	72	78		
	%	*100·0*		*89·3*	*60·5*	*39·0*	*35·1*				
30	v 2	1	2	13	11	5	4				
	vw, g	0	1	2	0	0	1				
	R	203	198	170	148	101	111				
	%	*99·0*		*82·9*	*58·5*	*49·3*					
25	v 3	1	1	19	11	9					
	vw, g	1	0	0	1	1					
	R	235	233	195	172	153					
	%	*99·1*		*82·3*		*64·6*					
20	v 3	0	3	6							
	vw, g	0	0	0							
	R	203	194	176							
	%	*100·0*		*86·7*							
15	v 3	1									
	vw, g	0									
	R	92									
	%	*96·8*									
10		2									

	10	15	20	25	30	35	40	45	50
Total of unmarried by age groups.	1206	1077	654	355	184	93	44	14	6
Total years lived.	5707·5	4327·5	2532·5	1347·5	692·5	342·5	145	50	
Number of marriages.	37	247	146	70	19	7	1	0	

v = married   vw, g = divorced and widowed

SOURCE: Essen-Möller, E. (1935) page 76, Table 20. See pages 76–86 of his original German text.

similar to the general population in most significant medical and social respects. He followed up 57 per cent of the town control group, and Makela appeared to have obtained 100 per cent response rate to his Bavarian sample. A preliminary analysis by age and admission, diagnosis, length of stay, and social class indicated that Essen-Möller's sample was representative of the clinical groups selected, when compared with data from Luxenburger's previous studies.

The analysis of probability of marriage improved on that of previous studies by taking into account the age distribution of the sample compared with that of Munich and Bavaria, as given in the 1910 and 1925 Censuses. Essen-Möller discovered a high proportion of single schizophrenics before first admission which did not appear to be due to the effects of war in the relevant years, while the manic-depressives appeared to be very similar to the corresponding general population. Unfortunately he complicated the analysis in a dubious manner by artificially increasing the number of married patients; it appeared that widowed patients had been admitted twice as frequently as married ones, taking into consideration the corresponding numbers in these marital status groups at risk in the general population, and Essen-Möller considered that for every married patient admitted there was probably one at home performing household duties and for this reason he doubled the number of married patients in each age group before calculating probability of marriage before first admission; in some age groups the number of married was trebled if there was a corresponding increase in the rate of widowed patients admitted in these age groups. Even after these corrections, he concluded that schizophrenic women marry at a significantly low rate before their first admission, when compared with women in the corresponding general population. TABLE 2 allowed, for the schizophrenic women, a retrospective analysis of the period before first admission, and demonstrated that low proportions married existed independently of age on first admission. For example reading across the fifth horizontal row from the top of TABLE 2 he gives within each square marital status categories and proportion single at each 5-year age group for schizophrenic women who became ill at 35–40 years. Reading across the row, from left to right, at age 15–20, 100 per cent were single, 89·3 per cent at age 20–25, 60·5 per cent at 25–30, 39 per cent at 30–35, and at admission age 35–40, 35·1 per cent were single. Comparing this cohort with *those admitted* at the earlier age of 20–25, reading along the eighth horizontal row from the top in TABLE 2, from left to right, 86·7 per cent of these were single on admission, which is not significantly different from the proportion given (89·3 per cent) for older patients at admission, when they were aged 20–25. Low proportions married were discovered at all ages in this clinical group even when patients were not admitted until long after the most likely age at marriage early in the reproductive period. This appeared to be evidence for Kretschmer's view, that pre-psychotic schizoid traits are generally of long-standing among schizophrenics. Essen-Möller considered that schizophrenics could be treated as a homogeneous group regarding the estimation of probability of marriage before admission; however, there was some clinical differentiation within this category in that hebephrenic patients exhibited a lower marriage rate than catatonic or paranoid patients. This would agree with Kallmann's findings on paranoid patients, but not those on catatonics.

Essen-Möller was the first to attempt a systematic analysis of post-psychotic marriage rates. Frequencies of marriage for each age after illness were converted into probabilities by the same formulae as those used in the pre-psychotic analysis (formula from Wicksell (1931), referred to on p. 86, Essen-Möller, 1935). Essen-Möller found that the rate for schizophrenic women after first admission was between one-third and one-ninth of that found in the corresponding general population (and for men of this diagnosis it was between a quarter and three-sevenths). Manic-depressive women also experienced a decline in their marriage rate to half of normal during this period, whereas the male rate in this group was not so low. These low rates were not just due to hospitalization, because psychotic probabilities calculated only for the periods spent outside hospital also show a reduction. There was a definite relationship between higher post-psychotic marriage rates and more favourable outcome of schizophrenic psychoses, and the deteriorated cases did not seem to marry at all in this period. In spite of an extension of Wicksell's method no definite statistical relationship could be found between age at onset of schizophrenia and post-psychotic probability of remaining single.

Essen-Möller's analysis of pre- and post-psychotic legitimate fertility was controlled for age at marriage, and duration of marriage and is therefore far superior to the work of all previous investigators. Considering the period before illness, for marriages contracted before 1904 when the German population was not generally practising birth control, schizophrenic women produced about half as many children as the controls, whereas the manic-depressives showed no significant differences. For marriages between 1904 and 1918 there was a reduction in fertility for both clinical groups of patients, as the general birth rate fell, and the fertility of schizophrenic women became similar to that of other groups.

By the time the general population was practising birth control, as shown in the fertility of marriages contracted between 1919 and 1927, all clinical groups showed a corresponding decline in birth rate but schizophrenic men lagged behind the general decline and exhibited a significantly higher fertility rate which could not be explained in terms of differential social stratification. Essen-Möller attempted to relate the pre-psychotic fertility rates to the time interval between age at marriage and age at admission, but found the numbers too small in each cell to make any conclusions possible. However, he did find that the birth rate in the year before first hospital admission was greater than would be expected (on the basis of an average birth rate calculated for all marriages of at least one year's duration, uncontrolled for residence). He concluded that it was likely that the pregnancy of a patient or of a male patient's wife led to postponement of hospital admission. This, of course, supported his hypothesis that selective social factors produce a biassed marital status structure on first admission, on the basis of which he had doubled the number of married patients.

When fertility after first admission was measured for pre-psychotic marriages, it was found that in schizophrenics the post-psychotic rate was 70 per cent of the pre-psychotic estimates. No such reduction was found in the manic-depressive group. Unfortunately Essen-Möller does not give the number of patients in each group. Although this took place of residence into account, he did not correct his estimates for age distribution at marriage. Taking post-psychotic marriages, no reduction in fertility was seen, not even in the schizophrenic women; these patients tended to be the healthier ones who only stayed in hospital a short while.

Essen-Möller further analysed the fertility after admission of pre-psychotic marriages by outcome of psychoses, as Rüdin and Schultz had tried to do, taking age structure into account, and found a reduction in the birth rate for cases who had not fully recovered. However, his follow-up was biassed towards the group who had been re-admitted, and he had no comparable data on recovered cases. Hence, no clear conclusions can be drawn regarding the possibility that post-psychotic fertility might increase, if hospitalization were shorter, as it has been in recent years with the advent of phenothiazines and other drugs, community care programmes, etc. Nevertheless, he does indicate that the reduction of post-psychotic fertility is not entirely due to hospitalization but exists independently of this.

Essen-Möller found that the illegitimate birth rate before illness was higher for those who eventually married than for those who never married. Before illness all groups showed a decline in the illegitimate birth rate as was probable in the general population, although no clear comparisons could be made, but after illness the illegitimate fertility of schizophrenics was reduced to half of what it was previously, whereas the illegitimate fertility of manic-depressives showed no such reduction.

We may summarize Essen-Möller's final conclusions as follows:

1. Schizophrenics reproduce themselves significantly less than the general population because of their low marriage rate and low age on first admission, and even when the corresponding general population practises birth control they would not replace themselves numerically. When there is no birth control the fertility of schizophrenic women is about a quarter of that found in the general population. In a modern society in which all social groups practise birth control the fertility of schizophrenic women is raised to half that of the corresponding general population.

    Essen-Möller considered that there was a need for systematic sterilization of schizophrenics, but that these would need to be identified about 2 years before first admission in order seriously to diminish their fertility.

2. Manic-depressives reproduce themselves at the same rate as the corresponding general population, in spite of their lowered marriage rate and higher mortality after first admission. This higher fertility is mainly explained by the later age of onset of manic-depressive psychosis.

In spite of Essen-Möller's attempts to control the relevant variables of age at marriage, duration of marriage, social class and place of residence in his analyses, the facts that his sample was not a random one and that he used the method of doubling the number of married patients in his series, render his findings difficult to interpret, and he has subsequently suggested (Essen-Möller, 1967, personal communication) that his correction for the under-representation of the married in hospital was overdone. His follow-up seems to have under-represented recovered cases, and his post-psychotic indices of schizophrenics are therefore probably too low.

Subsequent to Essen-Möller, Ødegaard (1946, 1953, 1960) in Norway and Erlenmeyer-Kimling, Rainer, and Kallmann (1966) in New York have undertaken follow-up studies, and Böök (1953) has also estimated total fertility of schizophrenics in northern Sweden.

Ødegaard (1953) analysed all first admissions to Norwegian Mental Hospitals during the years 1931–45; he calculated age-standardized admission rates for single, married, widowed, and divorced patients, and found that incidence of schizophrenia and manic-depressive psychoses was higher for the single than for other categories. The widowed did not show the high incidence reported in Essen-Möller's study and Ødegaard did not appear to agree with Essen-Möller's hypothesis that many married patients were protected by their families and are thus not admitted; instead Ødegaard considered that the statistics were in favour of the hypothesis that schizophrenics are discriminated against in 'marriage selection', and that the low proportion married before first admission was the result of their pre-morbid schizoid personality.

In a more recent paper (1960), Ødegaard took first admissions for 1936–55 and showed that it is the low probability of marriage before illness which accounts for the low total fertility of schizophrenics. He used census material to estimate age-standardized pre-psychotic marriage rates, ignoring for this purpose the widowed and divorced patients. The number of schizophrenic women married per hundred expected was 49·2 for 1936–45, and 56·6 for 1946–55 admissions (the rates for schizophrenic men being lower). In comparison the rates of manic-depressive women of 94·6 for 1936–45 and 91·6 for 1946–55 were higher, as would be expected on the basis of Essen-Möller's estimates.

In his analysis of pre-psychotic legitimate fertility, Ødegaard controlled only for age of patient at admission; he found the fertility of schizophrenics to be higher than that of manic-depressives. For example, for the earlier period schizophrenic women had 89·7 children per hundred expected, whereas manic-depressives only had 80·4, and for 1946–55 the estimate was 93·3 for schizophrenics compared with 83 for manic-depressives. There was also evidence that illegitimate fertility of schizophrenics was higher than that of manic-depressives. These findings do not agree with those of Kallmann on schizophrenics, nor those of Essen-Möller on the two clinical groups, although Ødegaard considered that his schizophrenics may be biassed towards the lower social classes who exhibit higher fertility than the rest of the population. Ødegaard gave an index of total (pre-psychotic) fertility in a 'reproductive rate' which he obtained by multiplying his marriage rate for each group by the fertility rate. Then he concluded that the total fertility of schizophrenics, as measured in this way, was about half of normal, and that of manic-depressives about three-quarters or more of the level in the general population.

In a twelve-year follow-up of 871 admissions to Gaustad Hospital, Ødegaard (1960) found some indication that the post-psychotic marriage rate was low but that the fertility of post-psychotic marriages was comparatively high. However, no analysis was made by diagnosis, as the groups were too small.

A current American survey in New York State compares marriage and fertility of a random sample of schizophrenics admitted during 1934–6 with that of a similar series admitted during 1954–6 (Goldfarb and Erlenmeyer-Kimling, 1962; Erlenmeyer-Kimling, Rainer, and Kallmann, 1966). A total of 1,677 of 2,706 index cases had been followed up until 1961, and either the patients or their close relatives were interviewed. The earlier series demonstrated the low proportions ever married as found by Myerson, Popenoe, and Dayton's earlier American results, 51·4 per cent of schizophrenic women were ever married compared with 65 per cent of women of childbearing age in the 1940 Census. The more recent cases demonstrated an increase in proportions married, as found in the general population during the intervening period, 62·2 per cent were married compared with 76·3 per cent in the 1954 Census. The fertility differential between schizophrenics and normal women seems to be disappearing; the mean number of children of all female schizophrenics' marriages was 1·8 for patients admitted during 1934–6 compared with the mean of 2·5 for the general population, whereas the comparative group admitted between 1954–6 had a mean family size of 2·5, exactly similar to that of the general population. (General population data based on all women of childbearing age were derived from Census reports.) The increase in fertility was very clearly given by Rainer (1968): Comparing the pre- and post-war samples the reproductive rate of schizophrenic women showed a relative increase of 86 per cent, whereas that of the general population only increased by 25 per cent. If the schizophrenics' fertility is expressed as a percentage of the general reproductive rate for women, the given increase raised the fertility of schizophrenics from 58 per cent of that of the general population in the 1934–6 period to 87 per cent of the general population in the later one.

In the post-psychotic follow-up, Erlenmeyer-Kimling and his colleagues took 1941 as the last date of observation for the early series, and 1961 for the

1954–6 admissions. They have not so far distinguished pre- and post-psychotic marriage and fertility, and gave cumulative indices, as those given above. Even after an 18–20 year-interval only 54 per cent of the 1934–6 series had married compared with 64 per cent of the later series. There was some evidence that post-psychotic births increased as a percentage of total births to patients in the post-war sample; this would be expected, owing to the development of community care; of the 473 cases in which hospitalization data was completed, 43·4 per cent of the earlier sample was continuously in hospital compared with only 20·7 per cent of the women in the later sample. It is not possible to review their findings satisfactorily until the final analysis of this research is published, in particular a separate analysis of fertility after admission.

Bean (1966) has produced some data which tend to support Erlenmeyer-Kimling and his colleagues' findings that the legitimate fertility of schizophrenics is not now significantly different from the general population. They followed up 164 female patients of mixed diagnoses 10 years after their discharge in the New Haven area of the United States, compared with a control group of non-treated women (matched individually for age, marital status, race, religion, and social class). There was no significant difference between the groups in mean family size. However, Bean's study was too small to give any reliable estimates between psychoses nor did he analyse fertility before and after admission.

A very recent article by Shearer et al. (1968) supports Erlenmeyer-Kimling, Rainer, and Kallmann's (1966) finding on the increased fertility of schizophrenics since the impact of community care. A five-year fertility rate of 17 per 1,000 women of reproductive age was calculated for in-patients in Michigan's six mental hospitals during the years 1935–9, compared with that of 61·2 for 1960–4, indicating an increase in the number of deliveries within the hospitals of 366 per cent. Of these deliveries, 63·6 per cent appeared to be schizophrenic mothers. The writers considered the increase to be an undesirable side-effect of the 'open door' policy in mental hospitals, and advocated giving effective contraception to female in-patients. Caution is necessary in interpreting such findings because it should be remembered that the quality of data on the pre-war series was probably far below that of the recent cohorts; higher mortality may have indirectly diminished the fertility of women in mental hospitals during the 1930s. Moreover, the writers had undertaken these estimates after a follow-up of recent patients, many of whom may have been re-admitted whilst pregnant which would add to the recent fertility rate; the misleading use of fertility rates has often been emphasized by demographers in favour of more controlled analyses of reproductive histories. Although an increase in the fertility of schizophrenic women appears likely, the author would suggest that the problem should be seen in perspective, namely in terms of the markedly reduced chance of marriage and increased frequency of separation and divorce, rendering the total fertility of the group lower than that of the general population, in spite of a lessening of fertility differentials.

Böök's (1953) study of schizophrenics in a rural area of northern Sweden is methodologically superior to all previous work, in that his calculations are based on the entire incidence, rather than just hospital admissions. He found 50 male and 35 female schizophrenics in the Swedish parish registers for the area between 1902 and 1949 and from hospital and district physicians' registers. The incidence of manic-depressives was too low for analysis. Böök considered that most of the schizophrenics were of the catatonic type, as elicited by examination of records and interviews where possible. Considering both pre- and post-psychotic periods, 73 per cent of female schizophrenics were married compared with 91 per cent of a control group of normal persons (matched for age and sex).

Böök's results are difficult to compare with others, in view of the unique nature of his area. He admits that the high proportion of married female schizophrenics may be the result of the shortage of young women in the area, and the fact that physical strength and resistance to the severe winters are more sought-after qualities in a wife than is usual in modern Western societies, so that schizoid personalities may not be so discriminated against in marriage selection in his area.

The mean family size of Böök's schizophrenic women was 5·96 compared with 4·68 in the controls. Böök therefore agrees with Ødegaard (1960) on the high legitimate fertility of schizophrenics, unlike Kallmann and Essen-Möller's findings on larger samples. There was almost no birth control practised in Böök's area owing to the prevalence of an orthodox puritanical religion (Laestodianism) and it is unlikely that the lower fertility of the controls may be attributed to a sociological bias towards middle classes.

There has been one Swedish estimate of the fertility of manic-depressives based on another detailed investigation of a small area. Stenstedt (1952) found 216 cases of manic-depressive psychosis in north-west Bohuslän (population 43,750 in 1948) who were treated between 1919 and 1948. He compared the marital status distribution of his probands with that found in the 1945 Census, and found no significant differences for the women when the χ^2 test was used (after onset the marriage rate of men suffering from this illness fell to about half the rate found in the general population). No significant fertility differentials were obtained nor were there any differences between the probands and corresponding general population data in the proportion of infertile marriages. Stenstedt's results therefore tend to agree with those of Essen-Möller's, and disagree with Kallmann's (1950) finding that manic-depressive twins over the age of 45 exhibited a lower fertility than his schizophrenic twins in this age group. It seems likely that the small size of this part of Kallmann's sample produced an unreliable estimate of the fertility of manic-depressives: there was a total of only 23 monozygotic and 52 dizygotic manic-depressive twin index cases. Stenstedt's comparisons with the general population depended on census data but his findings give further evidence that the fertility of manic-depressives is unlikely to be significantly reduced when compared carefully with that of the corresponding general population.

An interesting recent contribution to the literature is a study of marriage and fertility of psychotics attending an out-patient clinic in an Arab community during 1966 (El-Islam and El-Deeb, 1968). Sixty-five women of childbearing age, who were diagnosed as schizophrenics, showed a higher proportion single than that found for 68 manic-depressive women of corresponding age, and that found for a randomly selected control group of general medical out-patients of similar age, social class, and education and experience. The excess of single schizophrenics was found to be mainly among those of schizoid personality, which supports Ødegaard's (1946, 1953) hypothesis of the role of pre-morbid schizoid traits in reducing the chance of marriage of schizophrenics. An analysis of type of marriage of male schizophrenics demonstrated that there was a significant reduction in love marriages compared with arranged marriages in this clinical group, which indicated further that many schizophrenics lack the emotional warmth necessary for the normal pattern of love relationships. The fertility of schizophrenics also appeared to be reduced; 24 women who had been married for 1–9 years had a mean family size of $1 \cdot 1$ which was considered to be significantly lower than the mean of $2 \cdot 1$ for manic-depressive women, and $2 \cdot 2$ for 13 female controls, although the numbers are far too small to permit analysis by age at marriage and other relevant variables. An attempt was made to separate births to patients before and after onset of their psychoses, and schizophrenics appeared to have a lower proportion of children after onset ($15 \cdot 7$ per cent) than manic-depressive women ($37 \cdot 1$ per cent). However, it should be remembered that a large group of manic-depressives, whose illness began after the age of 50 and whose families were completed before illness, were excluded by the concentration of the study on women of childbearing age. These findings from an Arab community agree with those of Kallmann (1938) and Essen-Möller (1935) on the reduced fertility of schizophrenics in Germany and disagree with those of Böök (1953) and Ødegaard (1960) on fertility of patients in Scandinavia.

We may conclude that previous studies of this problem have either been too small to allow for adequate statistical analysis or that the larger investigations have either failed to control those variables known to influence fertility in modern Western societies in comparison with general population data, or they have been based on biassed samples or used dubious statistical methods. A large representative sample and follow-up is therefore necessary, which will analyse marriage and fertility before and after admission by rigorously controlled comparisons with general population indices. It seems likely that the probability of marrying of schizophrenics is reduced before first admission, and that considerable reduction occurs after discharge. Fertility of schizophrenics is a controversial issue: any difference from the general population will probably be slight, and mainly in the post-psychotic period. The probability of marrying among manic-depressives would seem to be the same as that found in the general population, although differentials may appear after first discharge. The fertility of manic-depressives is not likely to differ very significantly from that of the corresponding general population.

CHAPTER III

GENETIC AND SOCIAL RELEVANCE OF THE PROBLEM

GENETIC RELEVANCE

SCHIZOPHRENIA

THERE is now considerable evidence that schizophrenia is a genetic disorder, although environmental factors are often important in the production of a manifest psychosis. Geneticists are attempting to develop specific theories of gene transmission from basic empirical data on incidence of schizophrenia, increased morbid risks among relatives of schizophrenics, and the evidence reviewed in the previous chapter on reduced fertility of these patients.

Since the incidence of schizophrenia in England and Wales is estimated as 1·1 per cent of the general population, and Shields and Slater (1967) give a pooled estimate of 0·86 per cent from 19 studies throughout the world, it is particularly difficult to explain continuing high incidence in view of reduced probability of marriage and fertility. A brief review of the literature on the genetics of schizophrenia demonstrates the need for reliable estimates of fertility for geneticists to use in their calculations.

Twin Studies

Kallmann (1946) from New York produced the greatest amount of evidence for a genetic basis of schizophrenia in his analysis of 691 twin index families. He discovered that the uncorrected concordance rates for 174 monozygotic twins was 69 per cent, and for 517 dizygotic twins only 10·3 per cent. Kallman indicated that these rates were increased to 85·8 per cent for monozygotic twins, and 14·7 per cent for dizygotic twins when Weinberg's abridged method of calculating morbid risks among relatives was used. In simple terms, this was outstanding evidence for the importance of heredity in the production of schizophrenic disorders.

Subsequent twin studies have been unable to obtain such high concordance rates for monozygotic twins suggesting that the role of genetics in schizophrenia may not be quite so great as Kallmann indicated. Slater and Shields (1953) in England found the incidence of schizophrenia in monozygotic co-twins to be 68 per cent, Gottesmann and Shields (1966) found 50 per cent concordance, and Kringlen in Norway (1966) only 28–38 per cent. The latter estimate varied according to the concept of schizophrenia, and whether the sample was based on hospitalized cases or not. Subsequently Kringlen (1968) gave results from an analysis of all twins in the Norwegian birth register between 1901-30, involving 342 twins at least one of whom had been hospitalized for schizophrenia, manic-depressive psychosis, or reactive psychosis. He estimated that the maximum concordance rate for monozygotic schizophrenic twins was 31 per cent and felt that some forms of schizophrenia may well be determined by environmental rather than genetic factors. Regarding dizygotic twins, there has been slightly less disagreement (Slater and Shields (1953) found 18 per cent concordance, Gottesmann and Shields (1966) 12 per cent and Kringlen (1966) 5-14 per cent). The basic differential between monozygotic and dizygotic twins is the chief factor in maintaining genetic theories of schizophrenia, e.g. the higher percentage of both twins developing schizophrenia, when they are exactly the same genetically.

Criticism of Twin Studies

Rosenthal (1959) considered that the high concordance rates discovered by Kallmann and others could be due to factors other than genetic ones, in particular similar environmental influences. He stressed that problems of sampling from hospital admissions, unreliability of psychiatric diagnosis, problems of determining zygosity and statistical fallacies in the calculation of morbid risks all rendered definite conclusions impossible in this field (Rosenthal, 1961). From an analysis of Slater's twins, Rosenthal found more evidence that catatonic schizophrenia was inherited, than paranoid forms of later onset. In 1962 Rosenthal considered that the increased concordance rates for female compared with male pairs of relatives may also be explained in psychological terms of sex-role identification rather than on the basis of a sex-linked gene hypothesis.

Tienari (1963) in Finland found that out of a sample of male monozygotic twins born during 1920-9, who were alive in 1958, all 16 cases of schizophrenia were discordant, i.e. there was not one pair of twins who both developed schizophrenia. He had checked zygosity by serological methods, and felt that there must be other reasons than genetics for the high concordance rates found by Kallmann and previous investigators.

Since Kallmann's 1946 sample, some new data on this work were received by Shields, Gottesmann, and Slater (1967). Apparently Professor Kallmann had given Dr. Kety this new information in 1958, and the 1946 data were re-interpreted. It was decided that only 50 per cent of the 174 monozygotic twin pairs and six per cent of the 517 dizygotic pairs were concordant at the beginning of Kallmann's study. Other cases of schizophrenia were later discovered, and thereby increased the rates to the figures estimated above. Shields, Gottesman, and Slater (1967) found that new data on hospitalization and diagnosis exonerated Kallmann from criticisms of diagnostic contamination, i.e. more loosely diagnosing schizophrenia in a twin known to be monozygotic than in one known to be dizygotic. There was, however, some possibility that his particular use of Weinberg's age-corrected method of estimating morbid risks was not quite appropriate with monozygotic twins leading to an over-estimation of concordance. There seemed little evidence of faulty decisions regarding zygosity which could have biassed his findings, and the main reason for his high concordance rates was suggested to be the selection of samples of the most severe type of chronic, hospitalized schizophrenics. The value of the late Professor Kallmann's contribution to the genetics of schizophrenia was emphasized by the writers.

Increased Risks of Schizophrenia in Relatives

Estimates by Kallmann (1938) and subsequent writers have given widespread evidence for increased risk of schizophrenia among the families of schizophrenics. Pooled estimates given by Shields and Slater (1967) on the basis of fairly good agreement between countries are given below.

INCIDENCE OF SCHIZOPHRENIA AMONG THE RELATIVES OF SCHIZOPHRENICS

Sample	No. of studies	Incidence of schizophrenia
General population	19	0·86
Parents of schizophrenics	14	5·07
Sibs	12	8·53
Children	2	12·31
Uncles and aunts	4	2·01
Nephews and nieces	4	2·24
First cousins	4	2·91

Essen-Möller (1959) re-examined his 1935 data and stated that the low incidence (4 per cent) among parents of schizophrenics may be due to the reduced marriage and fertility in the previous generation of schizophrenics, i.e. 60 per cent of them are infertile. Rainer (1968) reports from the current survey in New York that some rates may be higher; taking 1 per cent as the risk of schizophrenia in the general population, he estimates a morbid risk of 14 per cent for sibs, 8–10 per cent for the child of one schizophrenic parent, and 53–68 per cent for the child of two schizophrenics. These estimates emphasize the relevance of genetics to the current survey on marriage and fertility.

Types of Genetic Theories of Schizophrenia

A recessive gene was originally postulated by Kallmann, on the basis of his 1938 study of Berlin schizophrenics. Subsequently Garrone (1962) was also inclined to this hypothesis, on the basis of a rather high gene frequency of 0·19, and an expectation of schizophrenia of 2·4 per cent in the general population. He considered that 3·6 per cent of the population were homozygous for the gene, with about 75 per cent of these becoming overtly schizophrenic in due course.

Other studies have considered that empirical evidence suggested a dominant gene responsible for schizophrenia. Böök (1953) in his study of a north Swedish isolate undertook a sophisticated genetic analysis: There was a high gene frequency of 7 per cent in his area (probably due to inbreeding), and supposing fertility to be 70 per cent of normal, he concluded that the dominant gene was of intermediate penetrance of 20 per cent in the heterozygote and 100 per cent in the rare homozygote. Slater (1958) postulated a monogenic theory similar to Böök's on the basis of his complex genetic studies in England. Slater then felt the gene was somewhere between the dominant and recessive types.

In their review of the field, Shields and Slater (1967) mention other genetic theories of schizophrenia such as those of Karlsson in Iceland, who postulated a dimeric theory involving a rare dominant gene of 0·03 frequency and a common recessive of 0·4 frequency being responsible for schizophrenia. Burch (1964) also suggests two common recessive genes as the basis of schizophrenia, their frequencies being between 0·34 and 0·50, but this theory involves other random events and is based on a specific concept of schizophrenia as an auto-immune reaction.

Geneticists have attempted to calculate the mutation rate for schizophrenia, depending on the particular theory of gene action preferred. Penrose (1956) took Kallmann's recessive hypothesis and calculated that with a gene frequency of 1 per cent in European populations, the proportion of schizophrenics in each generation which is due to fresh mutation is as low as 1 per cent of total incapacitated schizophrenic patients. Penrose had assumed from Essen-Möller (1935) that the fertility of schizophrenics was reduced to half of normal. Penrose's estimates do not seem to explain continuing high incidence of schizophrenia in view of this reduction in fertility.

The most important recent contribution to our knowledge has come from Gottesmann and Shields (1967) who suggest that a polygenic theory of schizophrenia may best fit the empirical evidence. This is particularly relevant to the current survey of fertility, because the theory allows not only the increased morbid risks found in families of schizophrenics which do not accord with classical Mendelian ratios, but also a slow response of incidence levels to negative selection, i.e. reduced fertility.

The main reason for departing from monogenic theories was the fact that in view of the reduced fertility, high mutation rates had to be postulated to account for continuing high incidence. Erlenmeyer-Kimling and Paradowski (1966) indicate that these high rates were much too high to be reconciled with Haldane's general estimates of human gene mutability (10^{-5}). Kishimoto (1957) for example, had undertaken a study of the population genetics of schizophrenia and using three different formulae to estimate mutation rates, 6 of 12 were between $3-5 \times 10^{-3}$. Erlenmeyer-Kimling and Paradowski suggest that an assumption of a genotypically heterogeneous basis to schizophrenia would allow mutation rates at different loci within the bounds

suggested by Haldane, which could make up for the effect of reduced reproduction. There may be some kind of polymorphism involving some advantage
to schizophrenics such as immunological mechanisms to make up for the
considerable disadvantages of pre-morbid personality and hospitalization
producing reduced fertility. Alland (1967) has pointed out that the search for
some kind of physiological advantage, such as resistance to stress, among schizophrenics would have to allow for the correlation of true incidence of schizophrenia in populations with variations in stress between populations. Possibly
the amount of penetrance could vary accordingly. This particular aspect of
research is obviously difficult because of the use of tranquillizing drugs in
schizophrenia, and the difficulty of obtaining untreated samples of patients. A
review of this particular aspect of the literature is beyond the scope of this
book. However, no physiological advantage has yet been definitely found
among schizophrenics. Recent research with families in Rainer's Department
suggests an increased reproductivity among the sibs of schizophrenics since
the Second World War.

Gottesmann and Shields (1967) suggest that their polygenic theory need not
involve the search for physiological advantages such as defence against stress
implied by Huxley *et al.* (1964). Gottesmann and Shields feel that a poly-
genically determined diathesis or predisposition to develop schizophrenia,
could be at more than one level, i.e. neuronal or cell-membrane, some genetic
influences may exert themselves early in development, others may only be
released in association with psychosomatic conditions or environmental
stresses. The polygenic theory allows explanation of the relationship between
severity of schizophrenia in twins and level of concordance in their co-twin.
Mild cases with good prognosis may have twins who do not reach the threshold
necessary to develop a manifest psychosis, although they may have schizoid
personalities. However, irrational and schizoid personalities would possess
some of the genes necessary to maintain the gene pool at the level required for
continuing high incidence. Falconer's technique (1965–6) for estimating heritability of the liability to schizophrenia was used by Gottesmann and Shields
(1967) and resulted in higher concordances among twins, although the polygenic
model permitted low incidences of schizophrenia among parents and sibs of
probands. The writers emphasize that the theory is only at its initial stage
(1967) because Falconer doubts the application of his method to monozygotic
twins, i.e. heritability becomes 51 per cent for mild schizophrenic monozygotic
twins which appears an over-estimation compared with the 17 per cent concordance rate found (Gottesmann and Shields, 1966). They conclude that
such research techniques which have appeared useful in the study of diabetes
may be profitably applied to the genetics of schizophrenia.

It should be emphasized that the polygenic theory of schizophrenia is still
in its initial stage. In 1966 Slater attempted a calculation to distinguish single
gene and polygenic effects by the study of expectation of abnormality on
paternal and maternal sides of relatives. Slater felt that if polygenic inheritance

was in operation, a more even distribution of secondary cases would be found when comparing maternal and paternal sides of families, than on a single gene hypothesis where there is only an increased frequency of affected relatives in one or other side of the family. Unfortunately, the calculation did not prove his hypothesis and increased frequency of affected parents or sibs was found on one side of the families even on the polygenic assumption. Slater hopes that more reliable empirical data on distant relatives or studies of families with three or more secondary cases could help eventually to distinguish polygenic and single gene effects.

Further Studies of relevance to Genetic Theories of Schizophrenia

Maternal age. In 1957 Goodman found that in a sample of schizophrenics selected from a psychiatric hospital in London the mothers of these patients had a significantly higher age at the birth of the patients than that found in the general population. This suggests that gene changes are more likely among the parents of schizophrenics and supports the view that genetic factors have a role in producing schizophrenic disorders. However, more recently Granville-Grossmann (1966) in another London sample, found no evidence for increased maternal age among schizophrenics, so that at present our knowledge is conflicting in this area.

Assortative mating. Although earlier applications of Mendelian genetics involved the assumption of random mating, the literature reviewed in CHAPTER II suggests considerable selection against schizophrenics in marriage. MacSorley (1964) and Nielsen (1964) also have found some evidence for assortative mating among schizophrenics. In Erlenmeyer-Kimling and Rainer's study in New York no increase in assortative mating has been found since the introduction of community orientated psychiatry: in their 1934–6 sample 0·9 per cent of schizophrenics married another patient of similar diagnosis, and in the 1954–6 sample the percentage of 1·1 per cent was probably not a significant increase. Erlenmeyer-Kimling and Paradowski (1966) suggest that assortative mating may be phenotypic but not genotypic if some assumption of genotypic heterogeneity underlying the schizophrenics is made; this could result in fewer children being affected by assortative mating than has been hitherto suggested.

AFFECTIVE DISORDERS

Twin Studies

There appears to have been less research on the genetic basis of affective disorders. The earlier work of Rosanoff *et al.* (1935) and Kallmann (1950) indicates 70–90 per cent concordance for this disorder in monozygotic twins.

Shields (1968) has recently undertaken an excellent review of psychiatric genetics, and with regard to affective disorders refers to the work of da Fonseca (1959) in Portugal. Considering endogenous affective disorders, 75 per cent of 21 identical co-twins, and 37·5 per cent of 39 fraternal twins like-wise had affective disorders. These estimates were not corrected for age and if concordance is restricted solely to hospitalized patients the rates become lower, i.e. 60 per cent for monozygotic twins and 31 per cent for dizygotic twins.

In 1963 da Fonseca undertook an analysis of 60 same sex twins with affective disorders attending the Bethlem Royal and Maudsley Hospitals. Some of these twins were monozygotic, some dizygotic, but da Fonseca found an increased frequency of somatic and psychosomatic syndromes among the co-twins such as asthma, peptic ulceration, certain dermatoses, and rheumatism. He called these 'affective equivalents' of a 'basic diencephalic disturbance underlying mood changes found in endogenous affective disorders'.

Theories of the Genetic Basis of Affective Disorders

Merrell (1951) postulated a dominant gene of incomplete penetrance because the increased frequency of affective disorders among relatives of patients was equal in sibs, parents, and children. Penrose (1956) accepted this hypothesis in calculating that one-seventieth of each generation of manic-depressives is likely to be due to fresh mutation, assuming fertility to be reduced by one-tenth as in Essen-Möller's study (1935).

It should be emphasized that the same questions of sampling, diagnosis and determination of zygosity apply to the above twin and family studies of affective disorders as well as to those on schizophrenics.

Relation between Genetic Basis of Schizophrenia and that of Affective Disorders

Kallmann (1946) in his study of twins failed to discover one case of a schizophrenic monozygotic twin in which there was manic-depressive psychosis in the other twin. The measurement of increased frequencies of psychiatric disorders in relatives has generally been confined to separate clinical samples of schizophrenics or manic-depressives, giving the impression of genetic independence of these two major functional psychoses.

However, Tsuang (1967) recently studied pairs of sibs both in hospital for mental illness and found that schizophrenia *and* affective disorders occurred *together* in sibs more frequently than could be accounted for by independent monogenic inheritance of each disorder. There is therefore some possibility that both schizophrenia and affective disorders could be largely polygenic and that, together with environmental influences, there may be some genetic overlap between the two types of disorders—as found perhaps in schizo-affective and paranoid-affective states.

In conclusion, the present survey of marriage and fertility should provide reliable estimates which are essential for geneticists to use in their calculations, especially any involving population projections of future incidence of schizophrenia or affective disorders. We must await a breakthrough in our knowledge of the exact genetic, or physiological basis of these illnesses, before the estimates given in this survey may be fully utilized. No attempt has been made to review Kety's (1966) assessment of the current work on the biochemistry of schizophrenia, nor other physiological studies which are beyond the scope of this book. The writer would, however, agree with Kaplan (1965) that there is a need for a multidisciplinary approach to the problems associated with the genetics of schizophrenia, and this also applies to affective illness. Longitudinal family studies involving psychological and sociological research into environmental factors in psychoses should be combined with methods of genetic analysis at the present stage of our knowledge.

SOCIAL RELEVANCE OF THE PROBLEM

Specific estimates of fertility of psychiatric patients should consider not only the intrinsic clinical condition, but also the impact of social change on the family, and the state of psychiatric and preventive medicine at the time of the investigation. Essen-Möller emphasized the fallacy of describing the 'fertility of the mentally ill' without due social and clinical classification. Kallmann's schizophrenics were treated during the 1890s when birth control was not practised in Berlin, when prognosis for mental disorders was poor, and long-term hospitalization characterized the lives of psychiatric patients. Today, in modern Britain, the problem requires a totally different approach. Rowntree and Pierce (1961 a and b) have indicated the spread of birth control to all social classes, and the use of tranquillizing drugs and other modern psychiatric treatments has resulted in community care of psychotics rather than long-term hospitalization (Brown *et al.*, 1966).

General Social Change

During this century, social change has altered the role of the family in Western societies. The emancipation of women has reduced the dominance of the male, and this has indirectly altered the treatment of female psychiatric patients. Since the earlier studies, the sexual needs of women have become more widely accepted, as Slater and Woodside's study (1951) suggested in respect of young married couples. Moreover, social and financial barriers have been removed from the English divorce courts, so that it is now easier to end unhappy marital situations (Rowntree and Carrier, 1958). Marriage today may be a less permanent contract than in the Victorian and pre-1914 era, and any discussion concerning marriage of psychiatric patients should take this into account.

The spread of birth control to all social classes may have lessened the need for sterilization of chronic psychiatric patients. If the healthy partner takes the responsibility for family limitation, this would avoid adverse effects of further pregnancies on the mental health of the female patient. However, there are some cases where religion prevents the use of appliance methods of contraception, and it is in these cases that a need for voluntary sterilization remains. A smaller proportion of female patients may be promiscuous and irresponsible, and sterilization would prevent the social problem of illegitimate children. Today it is not possible to generalize about sterilization of patients, and the specific problems in each case need very careful consideration.

Social Results of Developments in Psychiatric Medicine

Since the 1930s, developments in the treatment of psychiatric patients have resulted in shorter hospital stay and the care of psychotics in the environment of their families.

Most of the literature referred to here is based on schizophrenic patients, because this condition has the most chronic course and the worst prognosis. However, the more hopeful outlook found in recent studies applies to affective states and other clinical conditions. The change in social values towards accepting the mentally ill in the community is as relevant to our problem as specific clinical developments.

There is much evidence to suggest that prognosis in early schizophrenia is better than it has ever been. Before the Second World War follow-up studies supported Bleuler's (1911) concept that schizophrenics rarely recovered completely: 'By the term dementia praecox or schizophrenia we designate a group of psychoses whose course is at times chronic, at times marked by intermittent attacks, and which can stop or retrograde at any stage, but does not permit a full 'Restitutio ad integrum'.

Malamud and Render (1939) followed for 5 years 177 schizophrenic patients treated in an American State Hospital during 1929–36, and found 58 per cent unimproved and 10 per cent dead at the end of the study; in another American study Rennie (1939) was also pessimistic, in his 20-year follow-up of over 200 patients only 27 per cent were showing signs of recovery from schizophrenia.

But recent follow-up studies have shown that since the introduction of the phenothiazines in 1954–6, bed occupancy has fallen and prognosis has improved. Harris et al. (1956) found 45 per cent of schizophrenics living independently with no severe symptoms 5 years after their 1945–50 admission, and Brown et al. (1966) found 56 per cent living without severe symptoms 5 years after their 1956 admission. Nevertheless, there is a need for long-term follow-ups in order to estimate the real impact of modern treatment in schizophrenia and we should remember that Rennie found more deterioration evident after 20 years than after 9 years.

As a result of improved methods of treatment psychiatric patients now spend far more time at home than the patients selected by Kallmann and Essen-Möller. Brown has recently shown that early discharge policies regarding schizophrenics may cause considerable distress to relatives. Out of 339 schizophrenics admitted during 1956, between 19 and 33 per cent of relatives were experiencing severe problems associated with the patient during the final

6 months of their 5-year follow-up. Of 106 married schizophrenics, all the wives and half of the husbands reported multiple problems and adverse effects on their health. Divorce and separation were very frequent in Brown's sample; of those living with their spouse on admission in 1956, 31 per cent of the men and 12 per cent of the women had separated sometime during the 5-year follow-up, and considering both pre- and post-psychotic periods 44 per cent of the men and 27 per cent of the women who had ever married had separated from at least one marital partner. The corresponding percentage of divorces and separations in the general population should not be more than 12 per cent (Rowntree, 1964) for recent marriage cohorts. Brown considered that marital breakdown was three times higher than would be expected. However, their lack of control data for age at, and duration of, marriage, makes it impossible for the calculations to be so specific. Easier divorce and longer periods spent at home seem to have produced great instability and stress in the marriages of psychiatric patients. Thus the impact of early discharges on marital stability will receive further attention in the investigation proposed.

The problem of the probability of marriage and fertility of schizophrenics in particular is also sociologically relevant to psychodynamic theories of the causation of schizophrenia. The work of Lidz and Fleck (1960) suggests that the child develops schizophrenic ways of thought as a result of conflicts within the family. Farina (1960) considered that disturbance of role dominance in parents of schizophrenic patients produced the disorder. Frank (1965) suggests that longitudinal studies are needed to investigate the relation between parental conflict and the development of schizophrenia in children. From the opposite angle, there is considerable concern regarding the effect of psychiatric illness in the parent on the developing child (Rutter and Brown, 1966). Brown (1967) has reviewed the considerable literature on the family of the schizophrenic patient and the relevance of fertility to the problems involved should be emphasized. If further reliable indications are obtained regarding the adverse effects of the parent's mental illness on the child then patients should be advised, where appropriate, against bearing children for this reason as well as for the protection of their own health. In a recent review of the literature on the families of schizophrenics Brown has noted the tendency of investigators to base their theories on an insufficient amount of empirical evidence, and thus the exact significance of fertility to the above areas of research remains obscure.

It is very difficult to assess whether the social changes described above lessen or increase the total reproductive capacity of psychiatric patients in comparison with the general population. Essen-Möller (1935) indicates that in a population practising birth control the fertility of schizophrenics is higher when compared with the general population indices than in a population where no birth control is practised. This is presumably because he found that the fertility of male patients and their marital partners lagged behind the general decline in the German birth rate. However, we do not know at present the extent to which patients limit their families. With shortened length of stay in hospital, weekend leaves and a much smaller proportion of compulsory admissions perhaps fertility will be higher. To this we may add, as tending in a contrary direction, that tranquillizing drugs may repress sexual desire so that, even with more time at home, frequency of coitus may be lower than when the patient is well.

All these questions remain unanswered and the systematic collection of empirical data should precede further unsupported speculations on the differential fertility of schizophrenics and manic-depressives.

Part 2. Aims and Pilot Inquiries

CHAPTER IV

STATEMENT OF THE PROBLEM, AND PILOT INQUIRIES ON METHODS OF SAMPLE SELECTION

In 1963 the writer was awarded the Mapother Research Fellowship of the Medical Research Council in order to investigate 'The fertility of women now over 50 years of age who have previously had a psychotic illness not attributable to physical disease'. The psychoses referred to were schizophrenia, manic-depressive conditions and some mixed paranoid and schizo-affective states. Previous studies were considered to be inadequate [see CHAPTER II] and the following methodological criteria were considered necessary in the present inquiry:

1. A large random sample of psychotic women in order to estimate reliable fertility, and the effect of differential marriage rates on this.
2. The sample should be representative of the relevant psychoses in terms of age on first admission, clinical symptomatology and course of disease.
3. It should be possible to analyse pre- and post-psychotic fertility and there should be a follow-up of discharged and recovered cases for this purpose.
4. Adequate clinical and sociological data should be available for each patient from a source other than the patient, in order to analyse the results by the relevant variables of age at and duration of marriage, social class, religion, the course of the disease, etc.
5. Detailed data should be available for women in the general population of corresponding age, marriage date, social class, etc., either from official statistics or from a large control sample.

The pilot inquiries were to discover whether the selection of patients now aged 50 and over could result in a representative clinical sample.

THE FIRST PILOT INQUIRY ON SCHIZOPHRENICS, 1963

This aimed to discover whether a sample of schizophrenic women, aged 50 and over on recent admission, could be representative of all types of schizophrenia, including those forms which become manifest during early adult life. The records of Bethlem Royal and Maudsley Hospitals during 1957–9 showed that 64 women of this age and diagnosis were admitted during this 3-year period. Each patient had been diagnosed by the consultant within the categories 300·0–300·7 for schizophrenia in the *International Statistical Classification of Diseases*. Tabulation of the age on first psychiatric admission of these patients showed that 69 per cent of them were not admitted until they were aged 50 and over, whereas Norris (1956) showed that in London only 14–17 per cent of all schizophrenics are first admitted at this age. The method of sampling had resulted in a serious bias towards late onset of schizophrenia. Sixty-nine per cent of these patients had married and their mean family size was 1·88. Some reduction in fertility was indicated, but the numbers were too small to allow adequate comparisons with general population data. Moreover, all but 9 of the 64 women were paranoid schizophrenics, whereas 50 per cent of all schizophrenic women admitted during this period were non-paranoid cases, and therefore we may conclude that the method of sampling had produced a bias towards paranoid schizophrenia of late onset, and that forms of the disease which become manifest at an earlier age had been almost excluded. An alternative method of sampling was required in order to obtain a representative schizophrenic sample.

THE FIRST PILOT INQUIRY ON MANIC-DEPRESSIVES, 1963

This aimed to discover whether a sample of manic-depressive women aged 50 and over on recent admission would be representative of all forms of affective psychoses, and also to investigate the adequacy of the *International Statistical Classification of Diseases* (I.S.C.D.) and case file data for the present study.

A 50 per cent random sample of all such women was selected from the in- and out-patient records of the Bethlem Royal and Maudsley Hospitals for the years 1957–9. All 106 women selected had been diagnosed within the categories 301·0–301·2 for manic-depressive reaction in the I.S.C.D., their mean age in first psychiatric consultation was 53·31 (S.D. 13·55 years) and the sample did not appear biassed towards late onset when compared with the G.R.O. peak age of 55–65 for this disorder. However, analysis showed that 72 of the 106 patients did not become ill until after the age of 50, whereas previous studies have found a lower mean age of first admission (Stendstedt, 1952; $\bar{X}=39$ years). There is the possibility that most women, who experienced attacks during the childbearing period, had been excluded by the method of sampling.

The I.S.C.D. was most unreliable: cases of some organic bases had been included in category 301·2, and it was decided to sample from consultants' final diagnosis in the future, rather than from the classification.

Adequate data were obtained from case files on first admission, age at marriage, marital status changes, gynaecological histories, occupation of husband, religion of patient and hospitalization; but information was inadequate on birth control and incidence of specific mental illness in relatives.

The proportion married of all women aged 50 and over suffering from affective disorders during the period did not differ from that found in the corresponding general population of London (General Register Office, 1961b). The mean family size of the sample was 2·05 (S.D. 1·85), which appeared to be within normal limits, although analysis of patients and general population by marriage date and social class suggested a reduction in our cases which required further study.

It was concluded that the method of sampling women aged 50 and over suffering from manic-depressive conditions did not result in a serious bias in terms of disease onset as measured by first psychiatric consultation. However, it was decided to try alternative methods of sampling in order to make sure that women who fall ill of this disorder during the childbearing age are adequately represented. Official statistics were found to be adequate for comparison with case-file information, and these could be used in the main inquiry rather than to attempt to select a control sample.

SECOND PILOT INQUIRY ON SCHIZOPHRENIA, 1963

This explored the possibility of constructing a representative generation of schizophrenic women now aged 50 and over by selecting all admissions to a local mental hospital since 1916 of women born between 1900 and 1910, and whether a follow-up was possible of discharge and recovered cases who were treated 20–30 years ago during their childbearing period.

Since the Maudsley Hospital does not readmit chronic cases and serves no specific area it was not suitable, and a large chronic mental hospital which was within easy reach of the Maudsley Hospital was chosen for this inquiry. The map shows the catchment area of the hospital.

Unfortunately the hospital's record cards only went back to the 1940 admissions and discharges, and there was no sampling frame for the 1916–40 discharges except very large record books. Two samples of schizophrenics were selected:

1. All schizophrenic women born between 1900 and 1910 who were in the hospital during January 1963.
2. Ten married and 10 single women discharged between 1930 and 1934 were selected from old record books and a similar 20 were selected from the 1947–51 discharges in order to study follow-up problems.

First, the 161 chronic institutionalized cases obtained were not biassed towards late onset of schizophrenia: a mean of 34·3 years was obtained for single patients, and 39·8 for married patients. There was some possibility that mortality of earlier cohorts had produced some bias towards the more physically healthy schizophrenic. Only 46·6 per cent of these patients were married compared with between 70 and 84 per cent in the corresponding general population. The fertility of these deteriorated cases may be considered the lowest among schizophrenics, and a mean family size of 1·29 was obtained

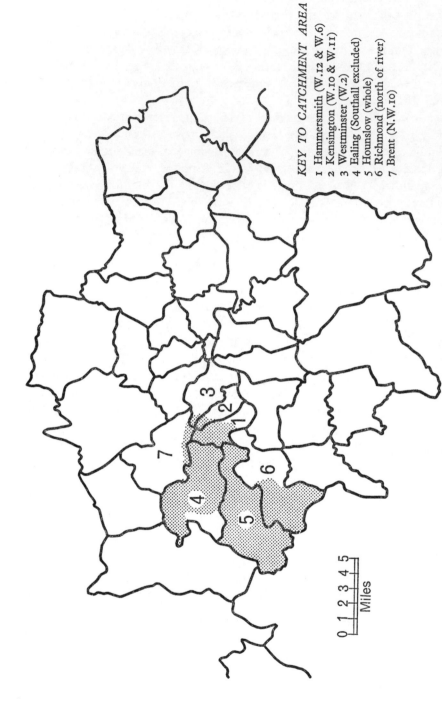

0 1 2 3 4 5
Miles

The catchment area of the Springfield Hospital in relation to the Greater London area.

(S.D. 1·4) which seemed to be between a half and three-quarters of that found in the corresponding general population of corresponding age and marriage date and social class. A high percentage of infertile marriages was found, i.e. 39·7 per cent compared with 21 per cent in the corresponding general population. These reductions in fertility could not be accounted for in terms of hospitalization, and appeared to occur even before first admission.

The follow-up of the 1931–4 discharges was impossible by postal methods and only 33 per cent of the sample were traced. Only 50 per cent of the 1947–51 discharges were traced. Almost half of the traced patients (7 out of 15) were dead at the time of follow-up, this bias may have been incurred by the reliance on hospital records in the follow-up inquiry.

It was not possible, therefore, to construct a representative generation of schizophrenic women who are now aged 50 and over by sampling retrospectively those admitted during their childbearing period and following them up by postal methods. More intensive follow-up methods were not considered possible by the writer in view of the large size of sample necessary for fertility analyses.

On the basis of the above pilot studies, it was concluded that it is not possible to obtain a representative sample of all schizophrenic women by sampling those now aged 50 and over, and therefore in the main inquiry we should sample women who are *now* of childbearing age. A similar sample of women suffering from affective illnesses should also be selected in order to make exact comparisons between these, the schizophrenics, and the corresponding general population.

CHAPTER V

THE AIMS OF THE MAIN INQUIRY ON WOMEN OF CHILDBEARING AGE

THE main inquiry aims to discover:

A. Whether there are any significant differences in the probability of marrying between schizophrenic women, women suffering from affective disorders and women of corresponding age in the general population.

B. Whether there are any significant differences between the fertility* of schizophrenic women, that of women suffering from affective disorders and the fertility of women in the corresponding general population.

In order to answer A and B on the basis of previous evidence the following empirical questions should be answered:

MARRIAGE

On the Probability of Marrying before First Admission for Psychiatric Treatment

Before their first admission, do schizophrenic women marry significantly less frequently than women of corresponding age, suffering from affective states, and do these clinical groups differ significantly from the general population in this respect?

Relevant Variables: Personality

Is there an association between pre-morbid schizoid personality and reduced probability of marrying in schizophrenic women before admission? Is there some parallel association between pre-morbid personality and reduced probability of marriage among women suffering from affective disorders?

Onset

Is the probability of marriage of schizophrenic women significantly more reduced among those experiencing a long period of symptoms before their first admission, compared with those patients experiencing a more sudden onset of their psychosis? Is there a parallel association between gradual onset and reduced chance of marrying among women suffering from affective disorders?

Age on First Admission

What is the role of age on first admission in reducing chance of marriage? That is, is the probability of marriage of schizophrenic women admitted before the age of 30 significantly more reduced than that of such women

* See page 4 for the definition of fertility in demographic terms which is used throughout this book.

admitted at a later age when they are compared with women of corresponding age in the general population during the calendar period before first admission ? Is there a similar association between age on first admission and reduced chance of marriage among women suffering from affective disorders ?

Mental Illness among Parents

Is there any relationship between probability of marriage before first admission and mental illness among the parents of the patients in either main clinical group ?

On The Probability of Marrying after First Admission

To what significant extent is the probability of marriage of both clinical groups reduced after first discharge when comparisons are made with women in the general population controlled for age and calendar period ?

Relevant Variables: Personality

Is the reduced chance of marriage after discharge in either clinical group related to problems associated with pre-morbid personality which may continue to exist after discharge ?

Age on First Admission

Does the age of first admission produce significant differentials in probability of marriage after discharge in either clinical groups, when comparisons are made with women in the general population, controlled for age and calendar period ?

Number of Admissions

Does the probability of marriage of schizophrenic women after first admission bear a clear relationship to number of admissions, i.e. the more admissions the greater the reduction in chance of marriage ? Is there a similar clear association among women suffering from affective disorders ?

Total In-patient Care

What is the role of hospitalization in significantly reducing probability of marriage in either clinical group ?

Course of Psychoses

Is the probability of marriage of schizophrenics who recover significantly higher than that of those who experience a more severe course of the disease ? Is there any relationship between course of illness and differential chance of marriage among women suffering from affective disorders ?

FERTILITY

Legitimate Fertility: before First Admission for Psychiatric Treatment

Is the fertility of schizophrenic women before admission significantly lower than that found in the corresponding general population, when the relevant

DMF

variables of age at, and duration of, marriage are controlled? Is there any fertility differential when women suffering from affective disorders are similarly compared with women in the corresponding general population?

Religion

What is the role of religion in producing differential fertility before first admission within either main clinical group?

Social Class

What is the role or occupation of the husband in producing differential fertility before first admission within either clinical group?

Education

Does the level of education attained by the patient bear any relationship to fertility before first admission within either clinical group?

Marital Happiness or Disruption

Is there any relationship between happiness or disruption of the marriage before first admission and fertility during this period within either clinical group?

Frequency of Sexual Intercourse

Is there any evidence to suggest an association between frequency of sexual intercourse and fertility before admission in either clinical group?

Fertility after First Admission

To what extent is the legitimate fertility of both clinical groups significantly reduced after first admission when compared with the fertility of women in the corresponding general population?

As in the case of the analysis of fertility before admission the role of religion, social class, education, marital disruption, and frequency of sexual intercourse in producing differentials within each clinical group will be assessed.

SPECIAL FACTORS IN FERTILITY AFTER ADMISSION

Hospitalization

To what extent are significant reductions in the fertility of schizophrenic women due to periods of in-patient treatment, when comparisons are made with women in the general population controlled for age at marriage, date of marriage, and duration of marriage? Is the fertility of women suffering from affective disorders less reduced because of shorter periods of in-patient care required in the treatment of these illnesses?

Course of Illness

What is the role of the course of the illness in significantly reducing fertility after admission among schizophrenic women, i.e. is the fertility of such patients who recover significantly higher than that of those who experience a more severe recurrent psychosis? Is there any parallel relationship between course of affective disorders and reduced fertility after admission?

Therapeutic Abortions and Sterilizations

What proportion of schizophrenic women are given therapeutic abortions and sterilizations? Does this reduce the fertility of this clinical group to any significant extent? Do a similar proportion of women suffering from affective disorders have therapeutic abortions or sterilizations, and is the fertility of this group reduced by these operations to any significant extent?

STABILITY OF MARRIAGE

Is the frequency of separation and divorce significantly higher among either main clinical group before their first admission than would be expected on the basis of other surveys based on the general population of women? Comparisons will control for age at marriage date and duration of marriage.

After first admission is there significantly increased frequency of separation and divorce among either clinical group when comparisons are made with women in the general population during this period? Is the proportion of separation and divorce higher among the schizophrenic women than among women suffering from affective disorders?

ILLEGITIMATE FERTILITY

Is illegitimate fertility in either clinical group significantly higher than would be expected in the general population of corresponding age? Are illegitimate births mainly before or after first admission? What is the role of psychological and social factors (i.e. such as race) among patients having an illegitimate child?

Additional Information

Is there any evidence for assortative mating among our patients? For example, how many of our female patients are married to male psychiatric patients?

Is the proportion of infertile marriages among either clinical group similar to that expected in a sample of women from the general population?

What appear to be the main causes of death among schizophrenic women and women suffering from affective disorders who die during their reproductive period?

Is there any evidence to suggest a significantly higher maternal age at birth of the patient among the mothers of the schizophrenic women than would be expected on the basis of general population data? Is there any parallel relationship between maternal age at birth of women later found to develop affective disorders?

Part 3. Methodology of the Main Inquiry

CHAPTER VI

METHODS OF SAMPLE SELECTION IN THE MAIN INQUIRY

IN order to answer the questions in CHAPTER V, it is necessary to select a large representative sample of women of childbearing age who have suffered from a schizophrenic or an affective illness.

HOSPITAL CHOSEN

It was decided to base the main inquiry on the mental hospital used in the second pilot inquiry on schizophrenics. The records of this hospital were known to be adequate for our purposes, and moreover all severe cases of mental disorder occurring within this hospital's catchment area were admitted, i.e. there was no selective admission policy which could bias our sample. By limiting the sampling to this hospital minimum time was wasted in travelling.

The map in CHAPTER IV gives the area within Greater London served by the hospital. TABLE 3 gives the total population of women of childbearing age for each borough which came within the catchment area, the proportions aged 15–30, and the proportions ever married. It should be emphasized that the catchment area, during the study, did not exactly follow borough boundaries, so that no exact estimate can be made of the total population served by the hospital. TABLE 3 indicates that there is a higher proportion of young women

TABLE 3

TOTAL POPULATION OF WOMEN OF CHILDBEARING AGE, PROPORTIONS AGED 15–29, AND PROPORTIONS EVER MARRIED, WITHIN THE CATCHMENT AREA OF THE HOSPITAL CHOSEN

Boroughs	N	Percentage aged 15–29	Total percentage ever married within each borough
Hammersmith	27,414	45·72	64·0
Kensington	53,411	54·04	45·2
Westminster	22,123	43·93	51·3
Acton	15,910	42·13	69·6
Brentford and Chiswick	13,560	42·23	67·3
Ealing	44,741	40·85	70·1
Heston and Isleworth	24,259	40·46	70·3
Twickenham	23,678	40·26	70·5

SOURCE: Census 1961, England and Wales. County Reports for London and Middlesex, H.M.S.O., General Register Office (1961b, and 1963a).

in the London Boroughs compared with that found in the appropriate areas of Middlesex: the lower proportions ever married in the London Boroughs are partly due to this differential age structure and perhaps to the fact that more single career women live in London.

TABLE 4 gives the socio-economic structure of the catchment area for occupied males. It shows that there is considerable variation within this area.

The London Boroughs of Kensington and Westminster and the Middlesex Borough of Twickenham contain a high proportion of professional people, whereas the Middlesex areas of Acton and Brentford contain more skilled manual workers. In CHAPTER IX there is a more detailed analysis of the socio-economic structure of the area in relation to the sample, which takes into account the occupations of women.

SAMPLING FRAME

The sampling frame used was the record of admissions: a card had been completed for each patient admitted giving name, sex, age, address, religion, date of admission, the consultant's initial diagnosis and the date of discharge, transfer, or death. The cards were filed in alphabetical order by discharge date. This record system was most suitable for the sampling of women of reproductive age who were suffering from specific psychoses.

DEFINITION OF PATIENTS STUDIED

The patients were defined as all women admitted to this hospital between 1 January 1955 and 31 December 1963, who were aged 16–49 years on their first admission during this period, and who were diagnosed by the responsible consultant as suffering from a schizophrenic or schizo-affective psychosis, and also all women in the same age group admitted between 1 January 1957 and 31 December 1963, diagnosed as suffering primarily from an affective disorder whether this be a manic condition, a depressive illness or a paranoid affective state.

Problems Regarding Diagnosis

On the basis of experience in the pilot inquiry on affective states (and in the light of conclusions reached by Lewis, 1934, 1944) no attempt was made to distinguish between psychotic and neurotic depressions. It should therefore be emphasized that the sample of affective states contained not only women suffering from manic-depressive psychoses but also those suffering from milder forms of depression. The sample is therefore not purely one of psychotics. However, all the women selected as affective disorders were suffering from severe disturbance of mood, either a depression or less frequently a hypomanic condition, and patients suffering solely from anxiety neuroses were excluded.

Although a complex definition of diagnostic categories was attempted by the writer, it was finally decided to accept the consultant's *last* diagnosis.

TABLE 4

SOCIO-ECONOMIC STRUCTURE OF THE CATCHMENT AREA OF SPRINGFIELD HOSPITAL: FOR OCCUPIED MALES ONLY

Proportions per 1,000 total economically active

	1	2	3	4	5	6	7	8	9	10	11	12	13	14	15	16	17
	Employers & managers in central & local government, large establishments, etc.	*Employers & managers in small establishments, etc.*	*Professional workers—self employed*	*Professional workers—employees*	*Intermediate non-manual workers*	*Junior non-manual workers*	*Personal service workers*	*Foremen and supervisors—manual*	*Skilled manual workers*	*Semi-skilled manual workers*	*Unskilled manual workers*	*Own account workers (other than professional)*	*Farmers—employers and managers*	*Farmers—own account*	*Agricultural workers*	*Members of armed forces*	*Indefinite*
LONDON																	
Hammersmith	21	44	4	22	31	154	16	32	322	143	126	38	0	—	1	4	41
Kensington	63	93	23	27	25	199	38	9	164	77	74	43	1	1	1	11	41
Westminster	72	115	24	46	58	222	73	7	112	65	78	31	2	—	2	51	43
All Greater London	50	97	21	44	52	185	59	14	167	100	111	40	1	—	1	24	34
MIDDLESEX																	
Acton M.B.	37	57	7	30	45	162	10	23	332	151	76	36	0	—	—	3	32
Brentford and Chiswick M.B.	44	64	8	36	51	179	16	25	309	127	75	34	—	1	1	5	25
Ealing M.B.	55	75	8	56	54	187	11	39	288	121	55	32	0	—	1	9	10
Heston and Isleworth M.B.	43	63	6	45	60	195	12	43	292	114	66	25	2	0	4	10	20
Twickenham M.B.	63	100	13	72	69	196	8	33	230	97	51	35	1	1	2	19	9

SOURCE: Census 1961 England and Wales, Occupation Industry Socio-Economic Groups. Separate reports for London and Middlesex, Table 5, page 46 (based on 10 per cent sample). General Register Office (1965 a and b).

Cases where there was a serious physical disease as well as a psychosis were analysed separately; all cases where the psychosis was the probable result of an organic disease of the central nervous system were rigorously excluded.

Unfortunately there was no record kept of patients who attended as out-patients but who were not admitted, and these could not therefore be sampled within the period allowed for the study. Their exclusion was probably more serious in the case of women suffering from milder affective disorders than it was in the case of schizophrenics, who generally required admission during the acute stage of the disorder.

A card was completed for each patient and a number allocated to her in numerical order of selection. The schizophrenics were selected first and then the women suffering from affective disorders.

SAMPLE SIZE

It was necessary to select a large enough sample to allow adequate statistical analysis by the relevant variables of marital status, age at and duration of marriage, age on first admission, social class, religion, and hospitalization. TABLE 5 gives the size of the sample by diagnosis and marital status.

TABLE 5

CONSECUTIVE ADMISSION SAMPLE OF SCHIZOPHRENIC WOMEN AGED 16–49 COMPARED WITH A SIMILAR SAMPLE OF WOMEN SUFFERING FROM AFFECTIVE STATES. N = 1,333

Consultant's final diagnosis	Marital status		
	Ever married	Single	Total
Schizophrenic disorders	449	362	811
Affective states	415	104	522
Total	864	469	1,333

Mr. N. H. Carrier, Reader in Demography at the London School of Economics, was consulted to determine whether the sample was large enough for the analysis required. It was decided that if a modified t test was used to test the difference between the mean family size of our cases and that expected on the basis of the corresponding general population, the sample would allow the detection of a 20 per cent difference which was not due to sampling fluctuations. The sample was also large enough for the detection of a 10 per cent difference in proportion ever married between our diagnostic groups and that found in the corresponding general population. It was impracticable for one person to cope with a larger sample, which would need a research team. However, all the women aged 50–69 admitted for schizophrenic and affective states during 1955–63 were also selected; there were 275 schizophrenics and 547 affectives in this group, and it was hoped to study these after the main inquiry on women of childbearing age in order to obtain more reliable estimates of marriage and fertility.

CHAPTER VII

METHODS OF COLLECTING DATA

DETAILED information on the marriage(s) and fertility of each patient was collected between 27 April 1964 and 31 August 1965.

INFORMATION OBTAINED FROM CASE RECORDS

After reading the clinical, social, and legal records of each patient, the questionnaire (given at the end of this chapter) was completed. This questionnaire was designed specifically for the proposed analysis of marriage and fertility, and care was taken in order to assess the periods of each patient's reproductive life before and after first admission.

In most records social histories were available from sources other than the patient, i.e. relatives and other hospitals. A note was made of the source of information from case records, and this was tabulated in the results. The nature of the information may be briefly described with reference to the questionnaire:

Page 1

Diagnosis: This was the last diagnosis given by a consultant at Springfield Hospital, the symptoms noted were those on which this diagnosis was made.

Marital status: Whether single, married, married apart, legally separated, divorced, or widowed.

Age on first psychiatric admission: This refers to the patient's first ever admission, whether to Springfield or to another hospital.

Pre-morbid personality: A note was made of this as described by the relatives, and in some cases an assessment was given by general practitioners. This information allowed division into three broad categories:

1. Schizoid (for example as described by Bowlby (1949)).
2. Prone to variable moods, eccentricities, or neurotic behaviour.
3. Apparently normal temperament.

Lack of interest in the opposite sex: This was obtained from the relatives' account of pre-morbid relations with men (or lack of them). (For single patients only.)

Hospitalization: This refers to any period of in-patient psychiatric treatment; in cases where there had been admissions to other hospitals information was obtained by post on diagnosis and length of stay. In this way data were obtained on any changes in the diagnosis of the patient, which would be used in the analysis.

Page 2

Note on the measurement of legitimate fertility: The questionnaire was designed in order to analyse mean family size by date and age at marriage and duration of the marriage, compared with that found in the corresponding general population. If patients had been married more than once, the fertility of their first marriages only was analysed. At the top of page 2 this information was noted at the time of the patient's first admission to Springfield Hospital.

At the bottom of page 2 the fertility of the patient during the period of her marriage *before first psychiatric admission* was noted.

In each separate assessment of fertility the expected number of live births was calculated (controlled for age at marriage, date, and duration of marriage in every case) from the Registrar General's Tabulations (usually Table PP in Part II of the *Annual Statistical Review for England and Wales*).

Illegitimate fertility: This includes births to single women which were not legitimized by subsequent marriage and births from extra-marital affairs.

Infertility and gynaecological treatment: Special hospital reports were written for if they were not available in the notes.

Occupation of husband and patient: The usual occupation was noted rather than the most recent, and this was coded in accordance with the Registrar General's Socio-Economic Groups. The husbands were also classified into the Registrar General's Social Classes (*G.R.O. Classification of Occupations*, 1960).

Age at end of full-time education: Referred to age of patient at leaving school, college, or university. Nursing and apprenticeships were not considered to be full-time education, and the school-leaving age was noted in this type of case.

Frequency of coitus: This could only be completed for married patients; a special note was made of any association between the patient's symptoms and disturbed frequency of sexual intercourse.

Marital relations (sexual and general): A note was made of whether the patient's marriage was described as happy by the husband or other close relatives. Details were noted of disturbed marital relations, especially if these were associated with the patient's illness.

Page 3

Hospitalization since marriage: For analytic purposes this was noted down separately from hospitalization whilst the patient was single.

Fertility after admission: The patient's fertility *since* her first admission was noted for all cases where there was more than one admission to a psychiatric unit.

Method of measuring mean family size after admission, taking into account hospitalization: This method was devised in order to answer the question in CHAPTER V, 'To what extent is any reduction in fertility after admission the result of hospitalization?' It was decided to see whether a reduction remained in fertility after admission when compared with an expected mean family size in the general population corrected for the loss of exposure to risk of conception which occurs during the patient's hospital stay. This correction was made by taking out of the expected fertility of the general population those births due to conceptions during those segments of marriage duration when the patients were in hospital. An example of this method is given on page 3 of the questionnaire:

This patient was married in 1947 when she was 18. She was first admitted in 1955 for 2 months, which means that she could not have any children during a 2-month period—9 months later in 1956. Thus in the ninth year of her marriage one-sixth of her fertility can be assumed to be reduced by hospitalization, and one-sixth of the general population fertility rate controlled for age at marriage, marriage date, and duration is 0·021. Similarly she was subsequently admitted in 1958 for 3 months, and 9 months later her fertility was reduced for that year by a quarter or 0·022 during the twelfth year of her marriage. Thus her total reduction in post-psychotic fertility due to hospitalization is only 0·04, i.e. as she only spent a short time in hospital the expected number corrected for this (0·33) is not much less than the uncorrected 0·37. In fact she has had one child, which is more than expected on the basis of the general population.

A modified t test may be used, and the actual births after admission for each patient summated and compared with the sum of the numbers expected in the general population. If there is a reduced fertility after admission the above correction factor will indicate whether this reduction is independent of the effect of hospitalization. If it is, then other causes of the reduction will be looked for, such as disturbed marital relations.

Onset: A note was made of the length of time between onset of symptoms and first admission, as given by the next of kin or the general practitioner.

Page 4

Mental illness in the parents of the patient, in the sibs and in the husband: Details were noted on any eccentricity in the relatives as well as specific psychiatric treatment received.

Data on sibs, marriage and fertility: This was discovered to be too vague to allow adequate analysis, and after the first few hundred questionnaires it was decided not to collect this data.

Mental illness of husband: Details were noted of any known mental or nervous disorder in the husband of the patient and in particular the diagnosis made if he had been seen by a psychiatrist.

Page 5

Leaves whilst in Springfield Hospital: Details were noted of the dates of periods at home for the purpose of correcting the total estimate of hospitalization used in the fertility analyses.

Between 27 April 1964 and 30 November 1965 questionnaires were completed on the entire sample (N = 1,333).

Page 6

This page was used to record the information obtained during the postal follow-up inquiry. Patients were not considered recovered unless very definite evidence was received about this from general practitioners, relatives, or patients' detailed letters.

Page 7

This was completed for the proposed analysis of probability of marriage in comparison with the corresponding general population (the probabilities were derived by computer, and not at the stage of collection from case records).

THE POSTAL FOLLOW-UP ON POST-PSYCHOTIC TRENDS

In the case of patients who had only been admitted once to Springfield Hospital, there was, of course, no information on the period after discharge. It was therefore decided to follow-up the entire sample (married and single patients) during the period allowed for the study, namely May 1964 to August 1966. Interviews would be too time-consuming except in a few cases where the patient had been re-admitted during this period, and therefore the follow-up was undertaken by post.

Method of Organization of the Follow-up

Cases discharged during the earlier years were followed up at first, i.e. 1955–6, 1957–8, discharges on the assumption that the greater lapse of time since these discharges would result in high non-response, and therefore more work would be needed to trace these patients.

First Stage of the Follow-up

For every discharged series the first stage of the follow-up was to check the appropriate electoral registers to discover whether the patients were still resident at the last address in the hospital records. In the case of those patients who had not moved a letter and a simple questionnaire were sent to the patient in order to obtain very basic data on marriage date (if applicable), live-born children, stillbirths, or miscarriages, husband's occupation and subsequent psychiatric treatment. If the patient did not answer within about one month the method of follow-up was as follows, i.e. as for cases who had moved:

(a) Relatives were contacted, whose addresses were on the hospital records, and they were asked either to complete the simple inquiry form of the patient or to send us the new address of the patient.

(b) The patient's last known general practitioner was written to explaining the nature of the research, and he was asked to give us the basic information on changes in marital status, fertility since discharge and subsequent psychiatric treatment (including routine drug therapy prescribed by general practitioners).

(c) Any other hospitals to which the patient had been admitted (these were known if they had written to Springfield requesting case notes). They usually sent us their own case notes for a short period, from which sometimes a new address helped trace the patient.

(d) Any friends or social workers noted in the case records were contacted if (a), (b), and (c) produced no positive response.

Second Stage of the Follow-up

In cases where all the above methods failed, there were three further possible methods of tracing patients, as suggested by Laurence (1959).

(e) The local executive councils for Middlesex and London gave us the names of new doctors of patients still living in their areas who had changed their general practitioners since their discharge.

(f) For patients who had moved outside the areas of Middlesex and London the National Health Service Central Register kindly traced their present doctors where possible (with the kind help of Dr. Benjamin and Mr. Rooke-Matthews). Information was also obtained regarding the death of some patients and the emigration of others.

(g) The Ministry of Pensions and National Insurance forwarded letters on to patients at new addresses if we sent them in a sealed stamped envelope. This method was only applicable to patients who had worked since their discharge.

The data obtained during the follow-up was used to fill in page 6, which was attached to the questionnaire for coding purposes.

The method of measuring family size after discharge during the follow-up was exactly the same as described for page 3 of the questionnaire. The fertility rates for 1965 were not known at the time of the follow-up study, and it was decided to measure fertility up to December 1964, rather than to guess at more recent rates. Births occurring after this date were not therefore counted in the actual numbers. In cases where the month of the marriage was not known, hospital stay after March 1964 was not included in the correction for hospitalization because it would influence fertility after December 1964, i.e. after the date on which we stopped measuring fertility. In cases where the month of the marriage date was known hospital stay in the last 9 months of the 1963–4 year of the year of the marriage duration was not included; for example, if the patient married in September any hospitalization from 31 December 1963 to 30 September 1964 was excluded from the correction. (This method was in accordance with the fact that the Registrar General measures fertility rates in *completed* years of marriage duration.)

Every attempt was made to avoid upsetting the patients and when single patients were written to, no mention was made of psychiatric treatment in case they had subsequently married and not told their husbands (there is the possibility of a marriage being declared null if within the first year it can be proved that one partner was subject to recurrent fits of insanity prior to the marriage and which was unknown to the other partner).

The follow-up involved a great deal of work, sometimes eight or nine letters were needed before a patient was traced. An analysis of response rates by diagnosis will be made in the results. Most patients, relatives, and doctors were very helpful indeed, and there were only two or three cases of serious objection to the inquiry.

Prop. No.

M.R.C. Springfield Hospital Fertility Survey

Patient's name	Last Hospital number	Date of birth		
Address:		Date of adm.	*at*	*yrs.*
		1st	2nd +	
		Last discharge		
Main symptoms in case notes		Diagnosis		
Marital status on 1st adm. during 1955–61				
Date of marriage		Age at marriage	*Pt*	*H.*

Date at end of 1st marriage

2nd or subsequent marriages

Age at 1st psychiatric adm.   Marital status then

Pre-morbid personality:
Lack of interest in opposite sex:

For 2nd + adms: marital status changes before and since 1st adm.

Ages between 1st and present adm.:

Hospitalisation when patient was single and for all single propositi:

Total number of admissions

Total length of hospital stay

Adm. no.	Dates	Hospital	Diagnosis

Page 2 of Questionnaire

Illegitimate fertility:

1st marriage date and age of pt	Marriage duration on 1st adm. during period	Actual number of live births since marriage	Expected number of live births

Stillbirths, with dates (*Note if illegitimate conception*)

Miscarriages, with dates (*Note if illegitimate conception*)
           Include therapeutic abortions with special note.

If marriage is infertile, any reasons given:

Notes on any gynaecological treatment including sterilisation

Use of birth control	*Before illness*	Husband	Wife
	After illness		

Occupation of 1st husband   Soc. class

Occupation of patient

Religion of patient   Pt's husband

Patient's age at end of full-time education

Frequency of coitus:

After first discharge

Pre-psychotic fertility:

Marriage date	Pre-psychotic years of marriage duration	Actual number of pre-psychotic births	Expected number

Note on marital relations.

Page 3 of Questionnaire

Hospitalisation since marriage:

Adm. no.	Dates	Length of stay	Hospital	Diagnosis

Total length of hospitalisation since marriage

Post-psychotic fertility: Method 2

Marriage date	Yrs of marriage duration	Actual No. of live births	Expected no.
1947 at 18	8–11th	1	0·37

Post-psychotic fertility: Method 3, effect of reduced exposure

Admissions	Periods when can have no children	Length of hospital stay	Marriage duration yrs	Gen. pop. duration— specific fertility rate	Fertility of gen. pop. during hospital stay
1955 2 mths	1956 2 mths	2 mths	9	0·122	$\frac{1}{6}(0·122) =$ 0·021
1958 3 mths	1959 3 mths	3 mths	12	0·089	$\frac{1}{4}(0·089) =$ 0·022

Expected no. of post-psychotic live births
corrected for hospitalisation $0·37 - 0·04 = 0·33$

Length of time between onset of symptoms and first admission:—

EMF

Page 4 of Questionnaire

If patient is in hospital, clinical condition now

If patient died in hospital, age and cause of death

Patient's father's occupation

Patient's mother's age at her birth   F's age

Patient's birth order

Mental illness in parents: form	When and where treated
M	
F	

Total sibs

Sibs' name in birth order	Age at death	Whether married and family size	Age at which lost touch with

Mental illness in sibs

Name	Form of illness	Where treated	Dates

Mental illness in husband

Page 5 of Questionnaire

Leaves whilst in Springfield Hospital: give exact dates

Admission No.	To	From	To	From	To	From	

Page 6 of Questionnaire

Information obtained by follow-up since discharge
Marriage: *Changes in status since discharges*

F.U. period: Pt aged   *to*   yrs

Post-psychotic fertility: follow-up of incomplete cohorts

Method 2

Marriage date	Yrs of F.U. marriage dur.	Actual no. of live births	Expected no.

F.U.:—Stillbirths, or miscarriages with dates

Method 3: F.U. of women under 50 on discharge, who have been admitted to other psychiatric hospitals

Admissions	Periods when cannot have children	Length of hospital stay	Marriage duration years	Gen. pop. duration specific fert. rate	Fert. of gen. pop. during subsequent hosp. stays

Expected no. of post-psychotic live births,
during F.U. period, corrected for subsequent hospitalisations

Final correction to expected no.—*for all adms*
hospital stays before and after F.U.

Note on illegitimate births since discharge.
Psychiatric treatment during the follow-up.
Clinical condition at time of follow-up, e.g. in hospital, dead, at home but on drugs,
   recovered, etc.

Page 7 of Questionnaire

Probability of remaining a spinster

Patient's reference number

Card number

Age on first psychiatric admission

Calendar year of first psychiatric admission

Calendar year of first discharge

Calendar year at end of observation

Whether we have above data

Expected probability of being single on first admission

Expected probability of remaining single from first admission to the end of observation

Expected probability of being single from first discharge to end of observation

CHAPTER VIII

STATISTICAL METHODS AND DATA PROCESSING

STATISTICAL METHODS: INTRODUCTION

THE basic difficulty of statistical analysis arises from the demographic hetero-geneity of the sample. In CHAPTER IV we saw how it was impossible to obtain a representative sample of schizophrenics by selecting those now aged 50 and over, and therefore the main sample is composed of women of all the child-bearing ages [CHAPTER VI]. Considering the variability by age on first admission, age on discharge, age at marriage, and duration of marriage, the sample of 1,333 patients is not large enough to permit subdivision into groups of women observed from the same age in the same calendar year for the same period, controlled for all the relevant independent variables. The major task of the statistical analysis was to eliminate the invalidating effect of these circumstances.

It was decided that the best method would be to calculate individually for each patient the equivalent normal woman's demographic behaviour, i.e. the probability of marriage of a normal woman of the same age, at the same time, observed for the same calendar period as the patient. Similarly, for each patient the average number of legitimate children that a normal woman would have borne was calculated, controlled for age at marriage, date, and duration of marriage. These indices of corresponding normal women were included on each patient's schedule, as described in CHAPTER VII.

THE METHODOLOGY OF THE MARRIAGE ANALYSIS

Quite apart from the influence of psychoses, the probability of a woman marrying within a certain period depends primarily on three demographic variables:

1. Her age at the beginning of the period.
2. The calendar year at the beginning of the period (in order to control for fluctuation in yearly frequency of marriage in comparisons with normal women).
3. The duration of the period.

To simplify, if these three variables took 20 alternative values, then together they could take 8,000 values and our sample of 1,333 does not permit splitting into demographically homogeneous groups. It was there-fore important to devise a mathematical analysis of maximum discrimina-ting power in relating the probability of marriage of each patient to that of a corresponding normal woman.

EXPERIMENTAL WORK TO DISCOVER THE APPROPRIATE MATHEMATICAL MODELS

In order to determine the appropriate mathematical models for the marriage analysis, experimental work was undertaken on two alternative models; in both models it was necessary to solve maximum likelihood equations by iterative methods on the London University Computer (Atlas). The accuracy of these methods was measured by Monte Carlo simulation. *For readers who are mathematically inclined, a detailed exposition of these methods is given in Appendix 4, Part A of the author's Ph.D. thesis.* Considering both models, let i be attached to each patient in the sample $i = 1$ for the first, $i = 2$ for the second, etc. Suppose that the (unknown) probability of the ith psychotic woman marrying in a specific period of her life is $Q_i{}^1$ and the equivalent probability of a normal woman of the same age marrying during the same period is Q_i. In the two mathematical models alternative forms of the ratio $R_i = Q_i{}^1/Q_i$ were considered, i.e. the ratio of the probability of marriage of a psychotic woman to the probability of marriage of a corresponding normal woman.

One-Parameter Model

In this model it is assumed that the *ratio* of the psychotic woman's probability of marrying to that of a corresponding normal woman is *constant* for all women in one group of the sample, e.g. the schizophrenics. For example, denoting this constant ratio as K, if it is the appropriate model, it would mean that if K was 50 per cent, and a corresponding normal woman has a 90 per cent probability of marrying in the particular period then our patient would only have a 45 per cent chance of marrying (i.e. 45 per cent = 50 per cent of 90 per cent).

Our sample was not large enough to enable a precise test of whether the actual circumstances approximated to those on which this model was based. However, women in the sample were grouped according to whether their equivalent normal probabilities were under 10 per cent, 10–20 per cent, etc., and the actual proportions of patients who married were calculated for each group. In spite of the appreciable margin of error, diagrams showed that when the ratios are plotted against the mean group values of the Qs (i.e. probabilities) in most cases the ratios were constant and that the one-parameter model was appropriate as far as could be told. In other cases the evidence suggested an alternative mathematical model.

Two-Parameter Model

In this model, it is assumed that the *ratio* of the psychotic woman's probability of marrying to that of a corresponding normal woman *varies* for example between different age groups. Using the same notation as in the previous model it is assumed that the ratio $Q_i{}^1/Q_i$ is a *linear* function of Q_i, $R_i = A + BQ_i$, where A and B are constants. If B is positive, this means that if the equivalent normal probability of marrying is large (e.g. 90 per cent) then the *ratio* of the psychotic's chance of marriage to that of a normal woman is larger than if the equivalent normal probability was small, say only 10 per cent. Suppose, for example, the ratio was 80 per cent when the normal probability, i.e. Q, was 90 per cent, but only 20 per cent when the normal probability was 10 per cent. To clarify the meaning of this model, if the probability of marriage of a normal woman was as large as 90 per cent, the probability of marriage of the corresponding psychotic would also be high: i.e. 80 per cent of 90 per cent = 72 per cent; whilst if the probability of marriage of a normal woman was as low as 10 per cent, that of the psychotic would be very low, i.e. 20 per cent of 10 per cent, only 2 per cent. In Appendix 4, Part A of the author's Ph.D. thesis, the maximum likelihood equations and their iterative solution are given, also for this two-parameter model.

The construction of graphs showed that where the one-parameter model was inappropriate, the two-parameter model seemed an accurate fit.

Analysis of Probability of Marrying by Independent Variables

It was not possible to control for all the relevant independent variables in our estimates, however the probabilities of marrying before admission were analysed within each diagnostic group (schizophrenics and affectives) separately by the following variables:

1. Pre-morbid personality (schizoid, moody, or neurotic, or normal).
2. Length of time between onset of symptoms and first admission (up to one year compared with over one year).
3. Age on first admission (under 30 and over 30).
4. Mental illness in parents (any form of such illness compared with none).

The probabilities of marrying after first admission were measured in two ways:

(a) After first admission until the end of observation, allowing for the effect of first hospital stay in reducing probability of marrying.
(b) After first discharge until the end of observation which excludes the effect of the first period in hospital.

The following variables were each separately taken into consideration in the analysis of probability of marriage after first admission and discharge

I. Personality (as above).
II. Parents' illness (as above).
III. Total length of hospital stay, i.e. all periods of in-patient care added together (short stay = up to one year, compared with periods of 1 to over 10 years).
IV. Number of admissions (one only, compared with 2–9).

V. Course of psychosis (recovered compared with not recovered at end of observation. Patients could be out of hospital but still in the 'not recovered' category.

The Methodology of the Analysis of Fertility

This presented more complex statistical problems, and no suitable mathematical models could be found comparable to those used in the marriage analysis. The method of measuring actual mean family size and the calculation of expected numbers in normal women controlled for age at and duration of marriage was described in CHAPTER VII. It was extremely difficult to compare the socio-psychological context of childbearing in psychotics to that of normal women. For example, a normal woman of 45 has been married for 20 years and she and her husband have had ample opportunity to have all the children they want, and they are extremely unlikely to have another. But a schizophrenic woman of 45 married for 20 years may have experienced long periods of hospitalization, and she may on discharge be excessively inclined to intercourse and with few inhibitions left, even promiscuous. There is the possibility that another child is more likely in these circumstances. On the other hand, continuous intake of a tranquillizing drug may diminish the sexual urge, so that patients on such treatment may be less inclined to frequent sexual intercourse, and for this reason another child could be less likely.

It is therefore not possible to compare the psychotic groups, lacking a clear relationship with normal women to provide the link. For each diagnostic group the total actual and expected number of live-born children was calculated three times: (1) for the marriage duration before first admission; (2) for the marriage duration after first admission, the expected numbers included the periods when the patients were in hospital; and (3) for the marriage duration after the first discharge, the expected number excluding births to normal women due to conceptions during the calendar periods when the patients were in hospital. Then any reduction in fertility, independent of the hospitalization effect, could possibly be detected.

Each diagnostic group was analysed separately for the effect of the following independent variables:

1. Social class of husband (non-manual occupation compared with manual).
2. Religion (Protestant and Jewish, compared with Roman Catholics).
3. Education (no further compared with some).
4. Hospitalization (up to one year compared with 1 to 10 + years).
5. Marital relations (happy compared with disturbed in any way).
6. Frequency of coitus (infrequent compared with three times a month or more).
7. No abortions required compared with cases needing at least one abortion or therapeutic sterilization.

The actual mean family size and standard error of each group, e.g. non-manual schizophrenics, were compared with the mean expected for corresponding normal women, and the ratio of the $\dfrac{\text{actual mean—expected mean}}{\text{standard error of the actual mean}}$ indicates whether there is a significant difference between patients and women in the general population controlled for age at and duration of marriage. In order to reach the 5 per cent significance level this ratio must be at least 1·96 (i.e. this is a modification of the t test). If the actual mean family size of the clinical group is less than would be expected on the basis of the general population, the above ratio will be a negative value, if the actual mean is high and greater than the expected mean, the ratio will be positive. In Appendix 4, Part B of the author's Ph.D. thesis, an example is given of this special fertility analysis directly from the computer output, for any reader who may be interested in further details.

It should be emphasized that such controlled comparisons are not possible between groups of patients of different diagnoses nor between patients having the same diagnosis but differing in other variables.

The Interaction of Independent Variables

Simple cross tabulations of independent variables were made by a separate computer programme as a preliminary step in assessing the interaction of the variables described above in the analysis of marriage and fertility.

DATA PROCESSING

Coding of Questionnaires

After the questionnaires had been completed a 10 per cent random sample of them was examined in order to decide upon the most appropriate coding frames for punched cards. At this stage it was not clear exactly what medium of analysis would be available and therefore in order to retain maximum flexibility a scheme of single punching was decided upon. A copy of the entire coding scheme is given in Appendix 3 of the author's Ph.D. thesis.

Page 7 contained the basic data for the calculation of probabilities of marriage, and in order to avoid chance human error, the 'normal' probabilities of marrying were calculated by programs on Atlas and punched into a third card on the L.S.E. I.B.M. 1440. Since computer analysis was necessary there was no need to duplicate information from the first two cards on to this third card.

The coding of the questionnaires took 9 months between September 1965 and July 1966.

Reliability Checks on Coding

Every column was given a 10 per cent check either by the original coder or by another coder. If more than one coding error was found the entire sample was checked for that code.

The coding of calculations of expected numbers and the corrections for hospitalization were also given a 10 per cent check. Information obtained on leaves at home whilst the patient was still being treated in hospital was used to correct the estimate of total length of hospital stay. This stage of checking the coding took 2 months from July to August 1966.

Punching

The coded questionnaires were punched on to cards during August–September 1966, each card was checked for punching errors.

Computer Editing

All the data was analysed on the I.B.M. 1440 at the London School of Economics and Political Science. Despite the precautions taken it was recognized that some errors could remain, and therefore a thorough editing process was conducted:

The following tests were made:

1. That the three cards existed for each case and were numbered Type 1, 2, and 3.
2. That in no column were there punchings for codes which could not legally appear.
3. Fifty 'logical consistency' tests, for example to check that a woman who had never married had always been coded as 'Not applicable' for legitimate fertility.

Appropriate details were printed out for cases failing each test, and the orginal questionnaires were examined to trace the error. The cards were then repunched and submitted to the tests again. Editing continued from September until the beginning of December 1966, and a substantial number of errors were detected and corrected.

In order to avoid errors in the analysis, it was arranged that whenever the survey cards were read into peripheral storage of the computer as a preliminary to analysis, the three cards per case should be checked every time that they related to the same case number and were in order, i.e. card Type 1, 2, and 3.

Part 4. Results

CHAPTER IX

CLINICAL AND SOCIAL STRUCTURE OF THE SAMPLE

TABLE 6 [p. 68] gives the clinical structure of the sample by age of patient on first admission, in comparison with corresponding data for England and Wales. The sample was biassed towards the younger age groups, which is an advantage in such a study of fertility in that the problems studied were currently of importance to the patients and their families. The affective sample was smaller than the schizophrenic sample because first admissions for the former group of patients are more frequent after the childbearing period.

Eighty per cent of the total sample were traced during the follow-up. TABLE 7 [p. 69] indicates that single patients were often more difficult to trace than married ones; 35 patients whose marital status on last discharge was not known were excluded from this table. TABLE 8 [p. 70] attempts to relate marital status to course of illness and shows how the single tended to stay in hospital and die more frequently than ever married, although our sample was too small to permit an adequate age specific analysis of this. These results tend to agree with those of Wing, Denham, and Munro (1959) who found that single schizophrenics stayed in hospital longer than married patients of this diagnosis. However, Brown and his colleagues (1966) found no correlation between whether schizophrenics had ever married and severe disturbance at the end of a 5-year follow-up. Unfortunately, there were no differences in our recovered group by whether the patient was ever married. The sample seemed clinically representative for the purposes of this inquiry on the basis of these tabulations.

SOCIAL STRUCTURE (MARRIED PATIENTS)

The proportion of patients married to men in non-manual and manual occupations is given in TABLE 9 [p. 71]; a high proportion in the manual group was found for each diagnosis. According to the socio-economic structure of the catchment area of the hospital, the average proportion of manual workers would be between 48 and 50 per cent when all the relevant boroughs on TABLE 4, CHAPTER VI, are combined. Comparative data for Greater London for males aged 22–39 give the manual proportion as 52 per cent and this decreases to 49 per cent in older men aged 40–59 (Glass, see REFERENCES). It therefore seems likely that our sample was biassed towards women married

TABLE 6

DIAGNOSTIC STRUCTURE OF SAMPLE BY AGE ON FIRST PSYCHIATRIC ADMISSION

(Age distributions compared with those for all admissions during 1959, N = 1,272)

Age on 1st admission†	Schizophrenia undifferentiated	Paranoid	Catatonic	Schizo-affective	Total schizophrenic	Distribution %	R.G. % Distribution	Affective disorders	Distribution %	R.G. % distribution* for manic-depressives	Total number of patients
16–19	62	4	3	8	77	9·67	8·61	20	4·2	2·99	97
20–9	250	21	21	24	316	39·7	31·17	147	30·88	19·0	463
30–9	162	61	11	28	262	32·91	37·55	170	35·71	38·56	432
40–9	51	79	2	9	141	17·71	22·66	139	29·2	39·45	280
Totals by diagnosis	525	165	37	69	796			476			1,272

* SOURCE: The Registrar General's Statistical Review of England and Wales for the year 1959, Suppl. of Mental Health, Appendix Table 24(i) for women of the childbearing ages, p. 78. (General Register Office, 1962).

† There were 61 patients whose age on first admission was not known, and who were therefore not included in this table.

TABLE 7

PERCENTAGE OF PATIENTS NOT TRACED DURING FOLLOW-UP BY DIAG-
NOSIS AND MARITAL STATUS ON LAST DISCHARGE

| | Per cent. not traced | | |
	Single	Ever married	Total sample
Schizophrenia undifferentiated	16·9	18·4	511
Paranoid schizophrenia	18·6	18·8	171
Catatonic schizophrenia	31·6	10·0	39
Schizo-affectives	25·0	9·5	69
Puerperal schizophrenia	100·0	31·3	20
Paranoid affective states	–	10·5	25
Manic-depressive psychosis: manic and hypomanic states	25·0	12·5	20
All depressive states	33·3	19·2	356
Depression with specified neurotic trends	15·4	27·8	49
Puerperal affectives	50·0	25·0	30
Total sample per cent not traced	19·6		1290

to men in manual occupations, as the proportion in this group was always over 60 per cent. The reasons for this bias could be:

1. That incidence of schizophrenic and affective psychoses for married women is really higher among women married to manual workers, as is found for all males of social class V admitted in England and Wales (The Registrar General's Supplement on Mental Health, 1957–8, General Register Office, 1961a).
2. That women married to men in professional and more middle-class occupations are not treated in chronic mental hospitals so that they are under-represented in the sample.

In order to see whether (1) was the case, it was decided to tabulate the socio-economic structure of female admissions for schizophrenia and affective disorders from a separate area of London. Camberwell was chosen because of the existence of a special register of all patients living in the area who had been admitted to both long-stay hospitals and university psychiatric clinics. This should also give some indication of (2) social bias according to type of hospital chosen for sample selection.

Camberwell is a more working-class area of London than some of the boroughs within the catchment area of the hospital chosen in the main study. Thirty-one per cent of occupied males in Camberwell were in non-manual occupations (1961 Census Occupation Industry and Socio-Economic Groups for London (General Register office, 1965a)), and TABLE 10 [p. 72] shows how there appears to be no bias towards the manual group in the schizophrenics but this sample was too small to permit any reliable comparisons. It was

TABLE 8

PERCENTAGE DISTRIBUTION OF FINAL CLINICAL CONDITION BY DIAGNOSIS AND MARITAL STATUS ON LAST DISCHARGE

Diagnosis	Marital status	Dead	In hospital	Discharged but not recovered	Discharged but not sure if recovered	Recovered	Not known	Not applicable
Schizophrenia undifferentiated	Single	9·4	20·0	15·8	14·7	16·6	23·0	0·4
	Married	3·4	12·0	17·7	27·1	17·7	21·1	1·1
Paranoid schizophrenia	Single	8·5	13·6	6·8	23·7	23·7	23·7	–
	Married	2·7	13·4	20·5	25·0	20·5	17·0	0·9
Catatonic	Single	5·3	5·3	15·8	15·8	21·1	36·8	–
	Married	5·0	20·0	15·0	25·0	25·0	10·0	–
Schizo-affective	Single	6·1	12·1	18·2	9·1	30·3	24·2	–
	Married	4·9	9·8	24·6	23·0	27·9	9·8	–
All affectives	Single	2·3	5·7	14·7	23·9	19·3	34·1	–
	Married	7·1	3·3	19·9	24·5	20·4	23·4	1·4
All diagnoses		6·0	10·9	17·8	22·4	19·8	22·4	0·8

TABLE 9

SOCIAL STRUCTURE OF THE SAMPLE OF EVER-MARRIED WOMEN ON LAST DISCHARGE: PERCENTAGE OF HUSBANDS IN NON-MANUAL AND MANUAL OCCUPATIONS BY DIAGNOSIS

Diagnosis	N	Non-manual %	Manual %
Schizo-undifferentiated	210	29·0	71·0
Paranoid	85	35·3	64·7
Catatonic	15	20·0	80·0
Schizo-affective	50	32·0	68·0
All affective states	265	36·2	63·8
Total	625	33·0	67·0

necessary to tabulate all ages of patients because of the small size of the area and women suffering from affective disorders formed a larger group and appeared more likely to be married to men in manual occupations when they are not treated at teaching hospitals. Unfortunately, at the time of the analysis, it was not possible to obtain a larger sample from the Camberwell Register.

On the basis of these rough comparisons it appears that the main sample may be slightly biassed towards women married to manual workers, and this could be due to the selection of a chronic mental hospital for sampling purposes instead of a teaching hospital, rather than to a real increase in incidence of psychosis among the working classes.

TABLE II [p. 73] gives the proportion of our single patients in non-manual and manual occupations by diagnosis. It is even more difficult to assess whether this is a sociologically representative sample from the catchment area, firstly because the G.R.O. have published no comparative data on single women by borough. There are crude figures of women in specific occupations by boroughs in the County Reports for Middlesex and London of the 1961 Census, but these do not give socio-economic groups. Glass (unpublished) quotes from Rotherham (1962) that in 1960 53 per cent of a random sample of women aged 22–39 living in Greater London were in non-manual occupations, which was in excess of the proportion non-manual found for the rest of the country. Yet in our sample over 70 per cent of single women appeared to be in non-manual occupations. This may be because the single women have a higher proportion in non-manual occupations than all women who are working or that patients and their relatives gave the best job they have ever done rather than the more usual occupation, which would result in some upgrading. Comparison with data from Camberwell [TABLE 12, p. 74] suggests that the proportion of single women in non-manual occupations appeared to be just over 60 per cent for admissions to a chronic mental hospital, and, as noted above, this borough is more working-class than some areas of the catchment area of our sample. The proportion of women in non-manual occupations rose in the affective group treated at teaching hospitals serving the Camberwell area to over 70 per cent as was found in our sample. A slight bias

FMF

TABLE 10

SOCIAL CLASS OF MARRIED* WOMEN (BY HUSBAND'S OCCUPATION) TREATED FOR SCHIZOPHRENIA AND AFFECTIVE PSYCHOSES IN CAMBERWELL, 1965-6, BY TYPE OF ADMISSION

	Type of admission								
	Chronic mental hospital			Teaching hospital			No admission—all out-patients		
Diagnosis	N	Non-manual %	Manual %	N	Non-manual %	Manual %	N	Non-manual %	Manual %
Schizophrenia	18	38·9	61·1	8	37·5	62·5	24	33·3	66·7
Affective disorders	66	21·2	78·8	72	33·3	66·7	332	26·8	73·2

* All adults on the Camberwell Psychiatric Register.

towards single women in non-manual occupations should not unduly influence the clinical and social importance of the results.

TABLE 11

SOCIAL STRUCTURE OF THE SAMPLE OF SINGLE WOMEN ON LAST DISCHARGE: PERCENTAGE IN NON-MANUAL AND MANUAL OCCUPATIONS*
BY DIAGNOSIS

Diagnosis	N	Non-manual %	Manual %
Schizo-undifferentiated	243	70·0	30·0
Paranoid	57	75·4	24·6
Catatonic	18	66·7	33·3
Schizo-affective	29	82·8	17·2
All affective states	78	78·2	21·8
Total	425	72·9	27·1

* Categories based on the Registrar General's Classification of Socio-Economic Groups, 1960 (General Register Office, 1960).

RELIGIOUS STRUCTURE

TABLE 13 [p. 74] gives the proportion Roman Catholic found in each diagnostic group: this varied between 19 and 36 per cent, according to marital status and clinical category. Glass (unpublished) gives a tabulation based on 2,671 women, in which only 10 per cent are Roman Catholic. Our sample appeared to seriously over-represent Roman Catholic women and in view of the significant role of Catholic doctrines in preventing the use of reliable methods of birth control, this bias could lead to an over-estimation of fertility of the patients.

ETHNIC STRUCTURE

TABLE 14 [p. 75] indicates that the sample is predominantly of British white patients but that there was quite a large group of non-British whites (n=191), who are mainly Polish and Southern Irish, and there is a group of 68 coloured patients.

In view of the over-estimation of Roman Catholics, which was mainly due to the large group of non-British whites, it was decided to analyse the results in two stages: (1) for all races combined; and (2) for British white patients only, in order to permit more reliable comparisons with general population data.

SUMMARY OF ASSESSMENT OF CLINICAL AND SOCIAL REPRESENTATIVENESS OF THE SAMPLE

1. The sample appeared to be clinically representative of the chosen diagnostic groups, although a slight bias was evident towards the younger ages on first admission.

2. Sources of social bias in such a sample of women were extremely difficult to detect but there appeared to be slight bias towards single patients in

TABLE 12

SOCIAL CLASS OF OCCUPIED WOMEN* TREATED FOR SCHIZOPHRENIA OR AFFECTIVE PSYCHOSIS IN CAMBERWELL, 1965-6, BY TYPE OF ADMISSION

Diagnosis	Type of admission								
	Chronic mental hospital			Teaching hospital			No admission—all out-patients		
	N	Non-manual %	Manual %	N	Non-manual %	Manual %	N	Non-manual %	Manual %
Schizophrenia	24	62·5	37·5	7	42·9	57·1	22	50·0	50·0
Affective psychoses	26	61·5	38·5	21	71·5	28·5	122	63·9	36·1

* All adults on the Camberwell Psychiatric Register.

TABLE 13

RELIGIOUS COMPOSITION OF THE SAMPLE: PERCENTAGE ROMAN CATHOLIC BY DIAGNOSIS AND MARITAL STATUS*

Marital status on 1st admission	Schizophrenics—undifferentiated	Paranoid	Catatonic	Schizo-affectives	Affective states
Single	33·1	31·0	36·7	35·1	28·7
Ever-married	19·4	28·3	23·5	23·6	26·7

* These percentages are based on a total sample of 1,250 Protestant, Roman Catholic, and Jewish patients and omit the small group of 75 cases of Hindu, Moslem, or no known religion.

TABLE 14

RACE OF PATIENT BY MAIN DIAGNOSIS

Race	Schizophrenic	Affective	Totals
British white	605	439	1,044
Non-British white	119	72	191
Indian	10	1	11
Chinese	4	–	4
Negro-Jamaican	32	15	47
Negro-African	10	–	10
Greek Cypriot	5	5	10
Others	2	3	5
Not known	2	1	3
Total, all races	789	536	1,325

non-manual occupations and patients married to men in manual occupations but this was not considered to be of importance.

3. Roman Catholics were seriously over-represented in the sample mainly because of the inclusion of Irish and Polish patients, and in order to eliminate racial variations it was decided to undertake a special analysis of the results based on British white patients only.

CHAPTER X

PROBABILITY OF MARRIAGE BEFORE FIRST ADMISSION

INTRODUCTION

THE analysis of probability of marriage before first admission produced significant differentials between schizophrenic women and women suffering from affective disorders. Important differential probabilities were also discovered within the schizophrenic group. Although experimental work had indicated that the two-parameter model would be appropriate for the analysis of the schizophrenics, the final results showed how the one-parameter model was more applicable to both clinical groups. As described in CHAPTER VIII, all probabilities of marrying were expressed as the ratio of the probability of marrying of a specific group of patients to the probability of marrying of normal women of corresponding age, observed during calendar periods identical to the patients.

In view of the bias in the sample towards Irish and Polish Roman Catholics, and the large group of coloured patients, the marriage analysis involved two separate stages: (1) analysis by independent variables of all races combined; and (2) a similar analysis of only patients who were British and white.

GENERAL RESULTS

TABLE 15 gives the general results for the schizophrenic group and the group of women suffering from affective disorders. Considering all races, the schizophrenic women were only $70\cdot4\pm2\cdot3$ per cent as likely to marry as normal women before their first admission, whereas women suffering from affective disorders did not differ significantly from normal women during this period ($97\cdot2\pm2\cdot1$ per cent). The analysis of British white patients increased the probability of marriage for schizophrenics before admission to $73\cdot4$ per cent of normal, presumably because in Britain this group is more likely to be selected for marriage than a group of women of other racial origins. The British white affectives showed no reduction in probability of marriage before admission.

ANALYSIS BY INDEPENDENT VARIABLES: PERSONALITY

Analysis by pre-morbid personality demonstrated significant differences within each clinical group [TABLE 16, p. 79]. (As noted in CHAPTER VII, information on personality was obtained from relatives via social workers and psychiatrists, and from general practitioners in some cases.) The findings were most

TABLE 15

PROBABILITY OF MARRIAGE BEFORE FIRST ADMISSION OF WOMEN SUFFERING FROM SCHIZOPHRENIA AND AFFECTIVE STATES: ALL RACES COMBINED COMPARED WITH BRITISH WHITE PATIENTS ONLY
(Probabilities expressed as a ratio of the psychotics' probability to that of corresponding normal women*)

	Schizophrenics				Affectives			
	Single	N Married	Probability	Standard error	Single	N Married	Probability	Standard error
All races combined	374	378	70·4	2·3	83	336	97·2	2·1
British white patients only	279	302	73·4	2·6	60	282	99·6	2·1

* One-parameter model (see Appendix 4 on Statistical Methodology) in the author's Ph.D. thesis.

important among the schizophrenics: considering all races, 159 who were reported as definitely having always been introverted and poor mixers were only 52.4 ± 5.1 per cent as likely to marry as normal women, which is significantly lower than the probability of marriage before admission of 88.5 ± 4.9 per cent for 121 schizophrenics who had always seemed normal to their relatives (for readers who are interested all significance tests are given in Appendix 5 of the author's Ph.D. thesis). Another interesting result is that a large group of 210 schizophrenic women who had been prone to variable moods and eccentricities, but who were not considered to be poor mixers, had a probability of marriage before admission of 77.4 ± 4.4 per cent which is significantly higher than that obtained for those of schizoid personality, and lower (not quite significantly) than the probability found for schizophrenic women of hitherto 'normal' disposition. These differentials were also clearly demonstrated in the special analysis of British white patients; in which the difference between moody patients and those of normal temperament appeared to just reach statistical significance at the 5 per cent level; 96 schizophrenic women who were British white and of 'normal' pre-morbid personality were almost as likely to marry as the corresponding general population of women (92.0 ± 5.3 per cent). However, schizoid traits produce a clinically and socially significant reduction in marriage before admission irrespective of racial origin.

The differentials by personality within the group of women suffering from affective disorders were not of the importance found in the schizophrenic group. Whether we take all races or only British white affectives, the only significant differential was that the small group of schizoid temperament had a reduced probability of marriage before admission (87.2 ± 7.9 for 42 British whites) compared with the high probability (107.7 ± 2.4) for those of hitherto apparently normal personality (81 British whites). This difference appeared greater than in the analysis of all races. However, it should be emphasized that the majority of women suffering from affective disorders had a similar chance of marriage before illness to that of corresponding normal women.

LENGTH OF TIME BETWEEN ONSET OF SYMPTOMS AND ADMISSION

Analysis by onset produced further significant differentials within the schizophrenics [TABLE 17, p. 80]. Taking all races combined, 181 schizophrenic women who experienced a gradual onset of symptoms for at least one year before admission were only 48.8 ± 4.7 as likely to marry as normal women, whereas 263 patients of this diagnosis whose illness was of a more sudden onset had a significantly higher probability of marriage (75.5 ± 3.9 per cent of normal women). This significant difference remained when British white patients were analysed, although both probabilities were slightly increased. No such differentials existed among the group of women suffering from affective disorders, probably because in this group pre-morbid personality change

TABLE 16

PROBABILITY OF MARRIAGE* BEFORE ADMISSION OF WOMEN SUFFERING FROM SCHIZOPHRENIA AND AFFECTIVE STATES BY PRE-MORBID PERSONALITY: ALL RACES COMPARED WITH BRITISH WHITE PATIENTS ONLY

| Pre-morbid personality | Schizophrenics | | | | | | | | Affectives | | | | | | | |
| | All races | | | | British white | | | | All races | | | | British white | | | |
	S	M	Prob.	S.E.	S	M	Prob.	S.E.	S	M	Prob.	S.E.	S	M	Prob.	S.E.
Schizoid	99	60	52·4	5·1	79	48	53·3	5·7	14	37	86·9	7·0	12	30	87·2	7·9
Prone to variable moods, neurotic	97	113	77·4	4·4	81	92	77·4	4·8	27	123	99·4	3·2	24	108	99·2	3·5
Normal	39	82	88·5	4·9	29	67	92·0	5·3	16	84	102·2	3·5	7	74	107·7	2·4

S = Single, M = Ever married

* Probabilities expressed as ratio of the psychotics' probability to that of normal women: one-parameter model.

TABLE 17

PRE-PSYCHOTIC PROBABILITY OF MARRIAGE* OF WOMEN SUFFERING FROM SCHIZOPHRENIA AND AFFECTIVE STATES BY ONSET AND AGE ON FIRST ADMISSION: ALL RACES COMPARED WITH BRITISH WHITES

| | Schizophrenics | | | | | | Affectives | | | | | |
| | All races | | | British white | | | All races | | | British white | | |
	Total N	Prob.	S.E.	Total N	Prob.	S.E.	Total N	Prob.	S.E.	Total N	Prob.	S.E.
Onset: length of time between onset of symptoms and admission												
Up to 1 year	263	75·5	3·9	198	78·8	4·5	167	93·0	3·6	129	96·5	3·7
1–5 + years	181	48·8	4·7	153	49·0	5·1	107	96·9	4·1	89	99·0	4·4
Age on first admission												
Under 30	369	61·0	4·0	282	65·3	4·7	139	94·1	4·9	107	92·9	5·7
Over 30	383	75·0	2·8	299	77·2	3·1	280	97·9	2·2	235	100·9	2·2

* Probabilities expressed as the ratio of the psychotics' chance of marrying to that for corresponding normal women: one-parameter model.

is not so disrupting to social relationships as the personality changes which accompany the onset of schizophrenia.

AGE ON FIRST ADMISSION

Considering schizophrenic women of all races, 369 who were admitted before the age of 30 were only $61 \cdot 0 \pm 4 \cdot 0$ per cent as likely to marry as normal women, whereas 383 such patients who were admitted when older were more likely to marry ($75 \cdot 0 \pm 2 \cdot 8$ per cent) when compared with normal women during the period before admission [TABLE 17]. This difference remained in the analysis of British white patients but it is then only just significant, and both probabilities increase slightly. Again, no important differentials were found among the group of women suffering from affective disorders.

MENTAL ILLNESS AMONG THE PARENTS OF PATIENTS

Probability of marriage before admission was also analysed by parents' mental illness. No significant differentials were obtained [TABLE 18]. Mental or nervous disorder among either or both parents would not appear to be related to probability of marriage in either of our main diagnostic groups whether we consider all races or only British white patients.

COURSE OF ILLNESS

We attempted to discover whether there was any relationship between probability of marriage before admission and whether the patients were recovered at the end of the follow-up [TABLE 18]. Patients were only classified as recovered if very definite evidence of this was obtained; if they still required tranquillizing or antidepressant drugs or any form of general practitioner or out-patient treatment or if they had died, they were grouped as 'not recovered' with patients who stayed in hospital. Within the group of schizophrenic women of all races the chance of marrying before illness appeared higher ($76 \cdot 0 \pm 5 \cdot 0$ per cent) for those 149 who recovered than for those 287 who did not ($67 \cdot 1 \pm 3 \cdot 9$ per cent), but this difference was not statistically significant and analysis of British white patients produced no important change in these estimates. Within the group of women suffering from affective disorders the opposite differential was obtained; taking British white patients only, 69 who recovered were $95 \cdot 1 \pm 5 \cdot 1$ per cent as likely to marry as normal women compared with the probability of $105 \cdot 2 \pm 3 \cdot 1$ per cent for 107 who did not recover. However, this difference is not significant, and it would appear that probability of marriage before first admission is not clearly related to course of disease in either clinical group.

THE INTERACTION OF SIGNIFICANT VARIABLES IN PROBABILITY OF MARRIAGE BEFORE ADMISSION OF SCHIZOPHRENIC WOMEN

TABLES 16 and 17 showed how the variables of personality, onset, and age on first admission produced significant differentials within the schizophrenics,

TABLE 18

PRE-PSYCHOTIC PROBABILITY OF MARRIAGE* OF WOMEN SUFFERING FROM SCHIZOPHRENIC AND AFFECTIVE DISORDER BY PARENTS' ILLNESS AND COURSE OF PATIENTS' PSYCHOSES: ALL RACES COMPARED WITH BRITISH WHITE PATIENTS ONLY

| | Schizophrenics | | | | | | Affectives | | | | | |
| | All races | | | British white | | | All races | | | British white | | |
	Total No.	Prob.	S.E.	Total No.	Prob.	S.E.	Total No.	Prob.	S.E.	Total No.	Prob.	S.E.
Mental illness in parent												
None	529	68·1	2·8	407	70·4	3·2	300	97·1	2·4	247	98·6	2·5
Evidence of any functional or organic disorder	129	70·7	5·8	113	75·3	6·1	56	103·4	4·5	53	104·3	4·2
Course of psychoses (for patients)												
Recovered	149	76·0	5·0	128	75·5	5·4	84	93·9	4·7	69	95·1	5·1
Not recovered at end of observation	287	67·1	3·9	233	67·4	4·4	124	105·0	2·8	107	105·2	3·1

* Probabilities expressed as a ratio of the psychotics' chance of marrying to that for normal women: one-parameter model.

and cross tabulation of personality and onset for this diagnosis indicated some interaction between these variables. An onset of over one year was experienced by 30·5 per cent of the schizoid group, compared with 27·8 per cent in the moody and neurotic group, and only 14·3 per cent in those schizophrenic women of 'normal' personality. Although these findings are very much as would be expected, i.e. they accord with the reduced probability of marriage in the schizoid group, and in those experiencing a long period between initial symptoms and hospital admission, the similarity in the proportion experiencing a gradual onset of over one year between the schizoid and the moody groups does not explain their significantly different probabilities of marriage. It would appear that the statistics summarize multifactorial determinants of behaviour, and that length of onset is not so important as the *kind* of onset which has not been measured. Probably the withdrawal and introversion of the schizoid group is far more shattering to heterosexual contacts than moodiness and neurotic trends for however long they occur. (The importance of the kind of onset is further demonstrated by the fact that affectives experiencing a long onset do not have a significantly reduced probability of marriage, unlike the schizophrenics.)

Cross tabulations of personality and age on first admission did not appear to demonstrate any significant interaction; nor did cross tabulations on onset and age; and more sophisticated analysis of the interaction of these variables was not indicated. Schizophrenics admitted before the age of thirty have a more significantly reduced chance of marriage before admission than those admitted when older, quite independent of the effect of pre-morbid personality and length of onset.

SUMMARY OF RESULTS ON PROBABILITY OF MARRIAGE BEFORE ADMISSION

The results on probability of marriage before admission may be briefly summarized, taking the more reliable analysis of British white patients:

1. Schizophrenic women were only 73·4±2·6 per cent as likely to marry as normal women before their first admission, whereas the women suffering from affective disorders did not differ significantly from the general population in the probability of marriage before admission.
2. Within the schizophrenics, those of schizoid temperament were only 53·3±5·7 per cent as likely to marry as corresponding women in the general population, whereas those of a more normal disposition had a significantly higher probability of marriage of 92·0±5·3 per cent. The women suffering from affective disorders showed no such significant differentials by personality.
3. Schizophrenics who experienced a long period of symptoms before admission were only 49·0±5·1 per cent as likely to marry as normal women, compared with the significantly higher probability of marriage

of $78 \cdot 8 \pm 4 \cdot 5$ per cent for those who had a shorter period between onset of symptoms and admission.

4. Schizophrenic women who were admitted before the age of 30 were $65 \cdot 3 \pm 4 \cdot 7$ per cent as likely to marry as normal women, whereas those admitted later had a higher probability of marriage before admission of $77 \cdot 2 \pm 3 \cdot 1$ per cent.

This finding was not paralleled in the group of women suffering from affective disorders.

5. Analysis of the interaction of variables suggested the importance of the interaction of schizoid personality and a long period between onset of symptoms and admission in reducing the chance of marriage of schizophrenics, and the importance of type of pre-morbid symptoms, rather than length of time in which they occur, was indicated by the data from both clinical groups.

CHAPTER XI

PROBABILITY OF MARRIAGE AFTER
FIRST ADMISSION

INTRODUCTION

THE basic method of measuring probability of marriage after first admission
was similar to the method described in the analysis of the period before
admission, i.e. probabilities were expressed as the percentage ratio of the
psychotics' probability of marrying to the probability of marrying of normal
women of corresponding age observed during identical calendar periods to the
patients, the one-parameter model was applicable in the analysis of the period
after first admission [see CHAPTER VIII]. This period was measured in two
ways: (1) from the first admission until the end of observation; and (2) from
the first discharge until the end of observation, in order to exclude the effect
of the first hospital stay on probability of marriage. As in CHAPTER X all races
were analysed together at first, and then patients who were British and white
were analysed separately, in order to control for racial variation within clinical
groups and in order to permit more valid comparisons between each main
clinical group and the general population.

GENERAL RESULTS

TABLE 19 gives the general results: during the period after admission
probability of marrying of 374 schizophrenic women was reduced to just over
one-third of that found for normal women, whereas no such significant
reduction could be detected among the 83 women suffering from affective
disorders. The smaller size of the latter clinical group is due to the fact that
most of them are married on their first admission, leaving only a small proportion exposed to the chance of marriage after admission. The clear differential is demonstrated between the schizophrenic women and the women
suffering from affective illnesses whether the period was taken from their first
admission or from their first discharge, and whether all races are analysed
together or whether patients who were British and white were analysed
separately. In both clinical groups, British white patients were slightly less
likely to marry than all races combined, which is the opposite effect to that
obtained in the analysis of the period before admission when British whites
were a little more likely to marry than the group of mixed races. The differences between the two analyses are sociologically insignificant and should
not obscure the main clinical and sociological findings, i.e. the marked
reduction in probability of marriage after first admission of schizophrenic
women.

TABLE 19

PROBABILITY OF MARRYING* AFTER FIRST ADMISSION OF WOMEN SUFFERING FROM SCHIZOPHRENIA AND AFFECTIVE STATES: ALL RACES COMBINED COMPARED WITH BRITISH WHITES ONLY

| Method of measuring the period after admission | Schizophrenics | | | | | | Affectives | | | | | |
| | All races | | | British whites | | | All races | | | British whites | | |
	Total No.	Prob.	S.E.	Total No.	Prob.	S.E.	Total No.	Prob.	S.E.	Total No.	Prob.	S.E.
After first admission	374	39·9	4·2	279	36·0	4·6	83	86·7	13·6	60	80·6	14·6
After first discharge	374	42·4	4·5	279	38·3	4·8	83	90·5	14·0	60	83·9	15·1

* Probabilities expressed as the percentage ratio of the psychotics' probability of marrying to that of corresponding normal women: one-parameter model.

ANALYSIS BY THE RELEVANT VARIABLES

Analysis was undertaken of probability of marriage after first admission by the relevant variables of personality, age on first admission, onset, number of admissions and total length of hospital stay.

Personality (as measured from reports covering the period before admission)

First, considering personality, significant differentials were obtained within the group of schizophrenic women, as shown in TABLE 20, 99 of those of schizoid nature were only $18 \cdot 1 \pm 6 \cdot 5$ per cent as likely to marry as normal women after their first admission, whereas a smaller group of 39 schizophrenics of apparently normal temperament were significantly more likely to marry during this period ($62 \cdot 4 \pm 14 \cdot 2$ per cent). Those 97 schizophrenic women who were prone to variable moods, and other neurotic traits, but were not withdrawn or shy, were $42 \cdot 4 \pm 7 \cdot 7$ per cent as likely to marry as normal women, which was a significantly higher probability of marriage after admission than that obtained for the schizoid patients of this diagnosis. These differentials exist when the effect of first hospital stay was excluded and are in the same direction as those obtained in the analysis of probabilities before admission and demonstrate clearly the crucial role of schizoid traits in reducing the chance of heterosexual contacts leading to the normal pattern of engagement and marriage. In the separate analysis of British white schizophrenic patients the same significant differentials were obtained between patients of schizoid and normal personality, but the differential between the schizoid and the moody and neurotic patients was no longer statistically significant (at the 5 per cent level). The British white schizophrenics showed a slight reduction in post-psychotic probabilities when compared with all races but this difference is too small to be of social importance.

TABLE 20 shows how women suffering from affective disorders did not exhibit any significant differentials by personality during the period after their admission: this is for two reasons; first because they are an older group and less are available for a post-psychotic marriage so that standard errors are very large and differentials difficult to detect; and secondly because social withdrawal and other schizoid traits are less frequent and less intense in this clinical group of women.

Age on First Admission

Age on first admission is a variable which produced significant differentials within the schizophrenic group during the period before admission but it has little effect on probability of marrying after first admission [TABLE 21]. Considering both all races together and British whites separately, after admission and after discharge, schizophrenic women admitted before the age of thirty were a little less likely to marry after admission than those admitted at a later age, but these differences were slight and statistically insignificant

GMF

TABLE 20

PROBABILITY OF MARRYING* AFTER FIRST ADMISSION OF WOMEN SUFFERING FROM SCHIZO-PHRENIA AND AFFECTIVE STATES BY PRE-MORBID PERSONALITY: ALL RACES COMPARED WITH BRITISH WHITES

| Pre-morbid personality | Schizophrenics | | | | | | Affectives | | | | | |
| | All races | | | British whites | | | All races | | | British whites | | |
	N	Prob.	S.E.	N	Prob.	S.E.	N	Prob.	S.E.	N	Prob.	S.E.
Schizoid												
After admission	99	18·1	6·5	79	18·4	7·0	14	131·1	44·4	12	135·6	43·6
After discharge	99	19·8	7·0	79	20·1	7·7	14	165·0	60·3	12	173·8	60·3
Prone to variable moods, neurotic, etc.												
After admission	97	42·4	7·7	81	35·7	7·9	27	62·6	20·2	24	58·1	20·9
After discharge	97	43·8	7·9	81	36·8	8·2	27	63·6	20·6	24	59·1	21·4
Normal												
After admission	39	62·4	14·2	29	56·4	15·6	16	114·2	25·7	7	104·4	33·1
After discharge	39	68·8	15·3	29	62·8	17·0	16	116·0	24·6	7	104·4	33·1

* Probabilities expressed as the percentage ratio of the psychotics' chance of marrying to that of corresponding normal women: one-parameter model.

and did not obscure the marked reduction in probability of marriage after admission in all schizophrenic women. The women suffering from affective disorders, who were admitted before the age of thirty also showed a tendency to a more reduced probability of marriage after admission when compared with patients in this clinical group, admitted at a later age, but they did not differ significantly from corresponding normal women in chance of marriage (at the 5 per cent level of significance).

Onset

The length of time between manifest onset of symptoms and admission does not appear to be related to probability of marriage after admission in schizophrenics; there is some slight evidence that women suffering from affective disorders experiencing a long onset were less likely to marry than others in this clinical group, but the numbers were too small to produce any significant differentials [see TABLE 21].

SPECIAL FACTORS IN PROBABILITY OF MARRIAGE AFTER ADMISSION

Number of Admissions

Analysis by number of admissions has produced very significant differences in probability of marriage within the group of schizophrenic women. Considering all races combined, TABLE 22 shows that 130 schizophrenic women who were admitted only once were $81·4 \pm 10·4$ per cent as likely to marry as normal women afterwards, whereas those 226, who were admitted between two and nine times had a significantly lower probability of marriage of $26·8 \pm 4·5$ per cent. This basic differential remains when probabilities after first discharge were measured, and in the analysis of schizophrenic patients, who were British and white. The women suffering from affective disorders demonstrated an insignificant difference in the same direction, but their probabilities were never as reduced as those obtained for schizophrenics. Moreover, TABLE 22 shows how there was only a small group of women suffering from affective disorders who were single on admission (and therefore available for marriage during the period afterwards) and who required recurrent admissions. The separation of British whites seemed to produce slightly more reduced probabilities after first admission in both diagnostic groups, but this in no way obscures the basic clinical differentials.

Length of Hospital Stay

There were 209 schizophrenic women of all races who required less than one year of total hospitalization, and these were $60·7 \pm 7·5$ per cent as likely to marry as normal women after discharge, whereas the group of 132 women of this diagnosis requiring longer hospital stay was only $18·1 \pm 4·9$ per cent as likely to marry as normal women after discharge [TABLE 22]. Schizophrenic

TABLE 21

PROBABILITY OF MARRIAGE* AFTER FIRST ADMISSION OF WOMEN SUFFERING FROM SCHIZO-PHRENIA AND AFFECTIVE STATES BY AGE ON FIRST ADMISSION AND ONSET: ALL RACES COMPARED WITH BRITISH WHITES ONLY

Independent variable	Schizophrenics						Affectives					
	All races			British whites			All races			British whites		
	N	Prob.	S.E.	N	Prob.	S.E.	N	Prob.	S.E.	N	Prob.	S.E.
Aged under 30 on first admission												
After admission	243	39·0	4·5	182	35·8	4·9	48	86·0	14·3	37	80·6	15·2
After discharge	243	41·2	4·7	182	37·9	5·1	48	89·6	14·7	37	83·8	15·7
Aged 30–49												
After admission	131	46·8	13·1	97	36·9	13·1	35	94·5	50·6	23	81·1	53·4
After discharge	131	52·0	14·5	97	41·2	14·6	35	101·9	54·3	23	84·8	55·9
Onset under 1 year												
After admission	124	35·0	7·3	91	35·1	7·9	41	90·5	19·4	27	80·3	21·9
After discharge	124	37·1	7·6	91	37·1	8·3	41	92·9	19·3	27	81·9	22·1
Onset 1–5 + years												
After admission	116	37·4	8·0	98	34·3	8·5	20	73·3	27·8	16	75·2	27·9
After discharge	116	40·4	8·5	98	37·2	9·1	20	82·2	30·6	16	84·5	30·7

* Probabilities expressed as the percentage ratio of the psychotics' chance of marrying to that of corresponding normal women: one-parameter model.

TABLE 22

PROBABILITY OF MARRYING* AFTER FIRST ADMISSION OF WOMEN SUFFERING FROM SCHIZOPHRENIA AND AFFECTIVE STATES BY NUMBER OF ADMISSIONS, AND LENGTH OF STAY: ALL RACES COMPARED WITH BRITISH WHITES

| Independent variable | Schizophrenics | | | | | | Affectives | | | | |
| | All races | | | British whites | | | All races | | British whites | | |
	N	Prob.	S.E.	N	Prob.	S.E.	Prob.	S.E.	N	Prob.	S.E.
Only one admission											
After admission	130	81·4	10·4	87	74·1	12·3	96·9	20·8	37	85·2	22·8
After discharge	130	87·8	10·8	87	80·1	12·9	99·4	21·0	37	87·4	23·2
2–9 admissions											
After admission	226	26·8	4·5	177	27·8	5·0	81·6	18·2	27	80·6	18·8
After discharge	226	28·4	4·8	177	29·6	5·3	86·2	18·7	27	84·5	18·4
Length of stay: under one year											
After admission	209	57·9	7·3	148	53·6	8·1	90·4	15·3	53	81·5	16·7
After discharge	209	60·7	7·5	148	56·1	8·4	91·8	15·3	33	82·6	16·7
Length of stay: 1–10 + years											
After admission	132	16·7	4·5	109	16·0	4·8	57·1	32·9	8	60·1	33·6
After discharge	132	18·1	4·9	109	17·4	5·2	67·7	38·1	8	70·1	33·5

* Probabilities expressed as the percentage ratio of the psychotics' chance of marriage to that of corresponding normal women: one-parameter model.

women who were British and white also clearly exhibited this difference whichever period (after admission or after first discharge) is taken. The women suffering from affective disorders demonstrated a similar differential to a lesser extent, but this was not significant owing to the small size of the group of 12 long-stay patients, and the resultant large standard errors.

COURSE OF PSYCHOSIS

Analysis by course of psychoses produced a differential in the expected direction: 66 schizophrenics of all races who recovered by the end of the follow-up were $40 \cdot 5 \pm 10 \cdot 0$ per cent as likely to marry as normal women, whereas 155 who did not recover had a lower probability of marriage after admission of $28 \cdot 6 \pm 5 \cdot 5$ per cent [TABLE 23]. Unfortunately, this difference is not significant at the 5 per cent level, mainly because of the small size of the recovered group in this sample, owing to the fact that no patient was considered recovered unless very definite evidence to this effect was obtained. Many patients who had been discharged for some time were not allocated to the recovered group unless information was obtained that they no longer needed any form of treatment. With a larger recovered group, it seems very likely that course of psychoses would produce significant differentials in chance of marriage after admission. The British white schizophrenics exhibited the same differential, the recovered were a little more likely to marry than the same group of all races, whereas the schizophrenics who did not recover appeared less likely to marry than the corresponding group of all races. However, the racial differences were too small to be socially important, *and it should be emphasized that the analysis of British white patients has merely confirmed more reliably the basic differentials abtained on all patients.*

TABLE 23 shows that the women suffering from affective disorders did not exhibit any significant differentials by course of psychosis, although those 18 who had not recovered appeared less likely to marry than those patients of this diagnosis who had, whichever period (after first admission or after discharge) was taken, and whether all races, or British whites were considered. It seems likely that a larger sample would detect a significant reduction in probability of marriage after admission of women suffering from recurrent affective psychosis, but that the reduction would not be as statistically and socially significant as that found for schizophrenics. It should be emphasized again that the proportion of women suffering from affective disorders who were single on first admission was very much smaller than that found for the schizophrenics, rendering the detection of differential probabilities of marriage especially difficult in the group of affectives.

Analysis of probabilities after admission by mental illness in the parents of patients indicated that this variable was not significantly related to probability of marriage in either clinical group.

TABLE 23

PROBABILITY OF MARRYING* AFTER FIRST ADMISSION OF WOMEN SUFFERING FROM SCHIZOPHRENIA AND AFFECTIVE STATES BY COURSE OF PSYCHOSIS: ALL RACES COMPARED WITH BRITISH WHITES

Course of psychosis	Schizophrenics						Affectives					
	All races			British whites			All races			British whites		
	N	Prob.	S.E.	N	Prob.	S.E.	N	Prob.	S.E.	N	Prob.	S.E.
Recovered												
After admission	66	40·5	10·0	58	46·5	11·2	17	93·0	33·0	14	96·4	32·6
After discharge	66	42·3	10·4	58	48·2	11·5	17	93·8	33·0	14	97·2	32·5
Not Recovered												
After admission	155	28·6	5·5	126	23·6	5·6	18	76·5	22·3	15	72·3	23·6
After discharge	155	30·7	5·8	126	25·5	6·0	18	82·3	23·4	15	78·0	24·9

* Probabilities expressed as the percentage ratio of the psychotics' chance of marriage to that of corresponding normal women: one-parameter model.

INTERACTION OF SIGNIFICANT VARIABLES IN PROB-
ABILITY OF MARRIAGE OF SCHIZOPHRENIC WOMEN
AFTER FIRST ADMISSION

The results show clearly that within the group of schizophrenic women those of schizoid personality and those whose illness is chronic were less likely to marry than those of a more sociable nature, and those who require less institutional care. These basic differentials were clinically, socially and statistically significant whether the period from first admission or from first discharge was taken, and whether all races or only patients who were British and white were analysed. Cross tabulation of personality, number of admissions, length of stay, and course of disease demonstrated considerable interaction between these variables.

First, considering personality, 18·9 per cent of patients of schizoid nature had five or more admissions compared with 17·4 per cent of these subject to variable moods and only 7 per cent of patients of apparently normal disposition. The tendency for the schizophrenics of schizoid nature to experience a more chronic course of disease is further demonstrated by the fact that 53·6 per cent of them had more than one year in hospital, compared with 49·9 per cent of the moody group and only 41·7 per cent of those schizophrenics of a more normal pre-morbid temperament. The main differences within the schizophrenic sample were between schizoids and normals: 17·4 per cent of the schizoids were in hospital at the end of the follow-up compared with 11·7 per cent of the normals; 9·2 per cent of the schizoids had died, compared with 5·5 per cent of the normal group; 17·2 per cent of the schizoids required out-patient or general practitioner treatment after discharge compared with 10·9 per cent of the normals and only 19·5 per cent of the schizoids were recovered compared with 26·6 per cent of the normals. Thus the interaction between schizoid nature and poor prognosis seems indicated, although the differences in proportions are not large.

The number of admissions of single schizophrenics was obviously related to course of psychosis: 84·4 per cent of the hospitalized group at the end of the follow-up had required more than one admission compared with 52·2 per cent of the recovered group. Total length of in-patient stay was also clearly related to final clinical state: 81·9 per cent of the single schizophrenics who were in hospital had required more than one year's in-patient treatment, compared with only 26·5 per cent of the recovered group. Length of stay was obviously related to number of admissions: no patients whose total stay was under 3 months had more than three admissions, whereas 52·4 per cent of those in hospital for 5–10 years had 4–9 admissions.

No clear interaction of age on first admission and course of psychosis was detected, although there were slight indications that schizophrenic women admitted before the age of thirty were less likely to recover (15·5 per cent) than those admitted at a later age (23·7 per cent), but further research is necessary to obtain more reliable findings. There was also some slight indication that those who experienced a long onset of over 6 months were more likely to have long periods in hospital but the differences were slight.

SUMMARY OF RESULTS ON POST-PSYCHOTIC PROBABILITY OF MARRIAGE

Taking the estimates based on British white patients, which permit more reliable comparisons with general population data:

1. After their first admission the schizophrenic women were only 36·0±4·6 per cent as likely to marry as normal women, whereas women suffering from affective disorders had no such significant reduction in probability of marriage.

2. Within the schizophrenics, those of schizoid nature were only 18·4±7·0 per cent as likely to marry as normal women during the period after admission whereas those prone to variable moods had a higher chance of marriage of 35·7±7·9 per cent, and those of apparently normal personality were even more likely to marry (56·4±15·6 per cent). No such significant differentials by personality could be demonstrated among the women suffering from affective disorders.

3. Schizophrenic women admitted only once were 74·1±12·3 per cent as likely to marry as normal women after admission compared with the significantly lower probability of 27·8±5·0 per cent of normal for patients of this diagnosis admitted between two and nine times. Schizophrenics whose total length of hospital stay was under one year were 53·6±8·1 per cent as likely to marry as normal women after admission, which is significantly higher than the probability of marriage of 16·0±4·8 per cent of normal for those schizophrenic women requiring longer periods in hospital. No such significant differences were detected among the women suffering from affective disorders, partly because of the smaller proportion of the group available for a marriage after admission and partly because of the less chronic course of these disorders.

4. Schizophrenics who recovered were 46·5±11·2 per cent as likely to marry as normal women after first admission, compared with the more reduced chance of marriage of 23·6±5·6 per cent for those who did not recover. However, this difference was not quite statistically significant. No such differences were demonstrated among the women suffering from affective disorders mainly because of the small size of the group and large standard errors.

5. There was some interaction between the variables of personality, length of stay and course of psychosis within the schizophrenic group; in particular those of apparently normal disposition whose chance of marriage after admission was higher were also more likely to have less admissions and more likely to recover than patients of a more schizoid nature,

and those prone to moods whose chances of marriage were lower. However, the data suggested that the factors of schizoid nature and chronic course of psychosis were each independently important in reducing the probability of marriage of schizophrenic women after admission.

CHAPTER XII

LEGITIMATE FERTILITY BEFORE
FIRST ADMISSION

INTRODUCTION

THE analysis of legitimate fertility presented more serious statistical problems than the analysis of probability of marriage. It was not possible to build suitable models linking the fertility of patients to that of normal women, and it seems likely that no model comparable to that found for marriage exists. The basic problem was the tremendous variation in the socio-psychological context of childbearing not only between psychotics and normal women, but also between the schizophrenic women and the women suffering from affective disorders and also even within each clinical group. It is not possible to compare the fertility of groups within each clinical category and it should be emphasized, in presenting the results, that the only reliable comparisons are between any specified group of patients and normal women, these comparisons being controlled for date of marriage, age at marriage, and duration of marriage. Since the most severe difficulties apply to the analysis of fertility after admission, examples to illustrate them are given in the next chapter. For readers who are especially interested, the statistical methodology of the analysis of fertility is described in detail in Appendix 4, Part B of the author's Ph.D. thesis.

Legitimate fertility was measured as mean family size controlled for age at marriage and duration of marriage, and the two main clinical groups were each separately compared with the general population, as described in CHAPTER VIII. The period before first admission was taken as all those years of marriage duration up to the date of each patient's first psychiatric admission. Children conceived during the 9 months before first admission, but born afterwards, were usually included in the analysis of fertility after admission. The mean family size of each group of patients was compared with that expected in the general population of women, and in order for there to be a statistically significant difference at the 5 per cent level the ratio of the Actual-Expected means to the standard of the Actual mean should have a value of at least two.

As demonstrated in CHAPTER IX, the sample incurred a bias towards Roman Catholic patients, and therefore in order to permit more reliable comparisons with the general population the analysis of fertility was undertaken in two stages; (1) for all races combined; and (2) for British white patients only (as in the analysis of marriage).

GENERAL RESULTS

TABLE 24 gives the general results for the period before admission. The fertility of schizophrenic women was reduced but this was only statistically significant when British white patients were analysed separately, i.e. 295 schizophrenic women, who were British and white, had on average $1\cdot36\pm 0\cdot07$* children before their first admission compared with $1\cdot54$ expected in the corresponding general population. However, this difference is too slight to be sociologically significant, unlike the clear differentials obtained in the marriage analysis. The 354 women suffering from affective disorders only showed a slight but insignificant reduction in fertility when the 301 British white patients of this diagnosis were analysed separately and their fertility before admission seemed very similar to that of corresponding normal women.

ANALYSIS BY RELEVANT VARIABLES

Religion

The variables of religion and social class produced the greatest differences in the period before admission [TABLE 25]. First, considering religion, the group of Protestant and Jewish schizophrenics had a reduced fertility which became significant in the 259 British white patients of this diagnosis who had $1\cdot33\pm 0\cdot08$ children compared with $1\cdot5$ expected. The smaller group of 75 Roman Catholic schizophrenic women of all races had a slightly increased fertility when compared with the general population, as one would expect owing to their doctrines against the more reliable methods of birth control, but this difference is not statistically significant. The Protestant and Jewish women suffering from affective disorders had a reduced fertility but this was a statistically insignificant reduction irrespective of racial origin, and as in the schizophrenics, the tendency to increased fertility in the Roman Catholics did not reach a significant difference from the general population. The differential fertility by religion of patient appeared to be in the direction one would expect from studies based on the general population, which have shown the lower proportion of Roman Catholics ever using birth control compared with Protestants of corresponding date of marriage. (Rowntree and Pierce (1961b) Addendum to *Birth Control in Britain*, Part I, Table 15.)

Social Class

Analysis by social class as measured by husband's occupation did not appear to produce any significant differentials when schizophrenic women were compared with the general population. All social groups of schizophrenic women had a reduced fertility, which became more reduced when the British white patients were analysed separately, i.e. when coloured patients and Roman Catholic Europeans have been excluded. The 83 women suffering

---

* The figure after the $\pm$ sign is always the *standard error* of the sample mean, in this chapter and in CHAPTER XIII.

TABLE 24

LEGITIMATE FERTILITY BEFORE FIRST ADMISSION OF WOMEN SUFFERING FROM SCHIZOPHRENIA AND AFFECTIVE STATES: ALL RACES COMBINED COMPARED WITH BRITISH WHITE PATIENTS ONLY

	Schizophrenics					Affective states				
	Actual mean family size	S.E.	Expected mean*	Ratio of actual-expected to S.E.	N	Actual mean family size	S.E.	Expected mean	Ratio of actual-expected to S.E.	N
All races	1·42	0·07	1·49	−1·03	369	1·64	0·07	1·62	0·34	354
British whites only	1·36	0·07	1·54	−2·51	295	1·60	0·07	1·64	−0·61	301

* Expected means are derived from the Registrar General's Annual Statistical Reviews for England and Wales, Table PP, Mean Family Size (average number of live-born children to existing women, married once only at integral marriage durations reached in the calendar year, by age at marriage and calendar year of marriage). (General Register Office, 1963b.)

TABLE 25

LEGITIMATE FERTILITY BEFORE FIRST ADMISSION OF WOMEN SUFFERING FROM SCHIZOPHRENIA AND AFFECTIVE STATES BY RELIGION AND SOCIAL CLASS: ALL RACES COMPARED WITH BRITISH WHITE PATIENTS ONLY

Independent variables	Schizophrenics					Affectives				
	Actual mean	S.E.	Expected mean*	Ratio of actual-expected to S.E.	N	Actual mean	S.E.	Expected mean	Ratio of actual-expected to S.E.	N
Religion										
Protestant and a small group of Jewish patients										
All races	1·37	0·07	1·48	−1·44	284	1·57	0·07	1·69	−1·65	245
British whites	1·33	0·08	1·50	−2·27	259	1·59	0·07	1·68	−1·18	253
Roman Catholic										
All races	1·61	0·17	1·41	1·20	75	1·81	0·18	1·51	1·72	79
British whites	1·79	0·25	1·63	0·62	28	1·71	0·22	1·49	1·03	45
Social class										
Non-manual										
All races	1·36	0·13	1·47	−0·80	89	1·45	0·12	1·73	−2·34	83
British whites	1·28	0·15	1·48	−1·39	72	1·52	0·12	1·68	−1·33	85
Manual										
All races	1·47	0·09	1·54	−0·73	205	1·74	0·10	1·64	0·96	165
British whites	1·40	0·09	1·58	−1·86	166	1·67	0·11	1·66	0·14	141

* Expected means controlled for age at marriage and duration of marriage derived from the Registrar General's Annual Statistical Reviews for England and Wales, Table PP.

from affective disorders who were married to men in non-manual occupations demonstrated a significantly reduced fertility when all races were compared with normal women, but the difference of just over a quarter of a child (0·28) was really too small to be of real sociological importance. The women suffering from affective disorders who were married to men in manual occupations had a slightly increased fertility, and it would appear that the clinical groups demonstrate the usual fertility differentials by social class found in the general population.

OTHER VARIABLES

Education of Patient, Marital Relations, and Frequency of Sexual Intercourse

Further analysis of fertility before admission by educational level reached by the patient, marital relations, and frequency of sexual intercourse produced results of little social importance. TABLE 26 shows how all groups of schizophrenic women had a reduced fertility which was statistically insignificant, whether all races were analysed together or whether British white patients only were considered. The only differential to almost reach the 5 per cent significance level was in the small group of 49 British white schizophrenics who were known to have infrequent intercourse; they only had $1·18 \pm 0·17$ children compared with $1·49$ expected in the corresponding general population. The women suffering from affective disorders did not appear to differ significantly from the general population, whether all races or only British white patients of this diagnosis were analysed by these variables [TABLE 26].

Therapeutic Abortions and Sterilizations

An attempt was made to relate fertility before admission to whether the patients had ever had subsequent abortions or sterilizations. The group of 280 British white schizophrenic women who had never received such treatment had a significantly reduced fertility, i.e. they had a mean family size of $1·33 \pm 0·07$ compared with $1·54$ expected; the small group of 14 such British white patients requiring this gynaecological treatment had an increased fertility of $2·14 \pm 0·44$ compared with $1·63$ expected, but this difference was not socially nor statistically at the 5 per cent level. Again, the women suffering from affective disorders did not appear to differ significantly from the general population when analysed by this variable. The group of 281 women suffering from affective disorders who were British and white, and who had never received such treatment had a mean family size of $1·57 \pm 0·07$ compared with $1·65$ expected. In comparison, 14 British white women in this clinical group who had therapeutic abortions or sterilizations had a mean family size before admission of $2·36 \pm 0·52$ compared with a lower mean of $1·71$ expected. The increased fertility of patients in each clinical group receiving such treatment would probably become significantly greater than that expected in the general population of corresponding age at marriage and duration of marriage, if large enough series of such special gynaecological patients could be selected.

TABLE 26

LEGITIMATE FERTILITY BEFORE ADMISSION OF WOMEN SUFFERING FROM SCHIZOPHRENIA AND AFFECTIVE DISORDERS BY EDUCATION, MARITAL RELATIONS, AND FREQUENCY OF SEXUAL INTERCOURSE: ALL RACES COMPARED WITH BRITISH WHITES

Independent variables	Schizophrenics					Affectives				
	Actual mean	S.E.	Expected mean*	Ratio of actual-expected to S.E.	N	Actual mean	S.E.	Expected mean	Ratio of actual-expected to S.E.	N
Education of patient										
No further education										
All races	1·41	0·19	1·51	-1·09	210	1·62	0·09	1·66	-0·44	244
British whites	1·37	0·10	1·53	-1·70	174	1·58	0·08	1·67	-1·11	225
Some further education										
All races	1·33	0·16	1·34	-0·09	61	1·34	0·14	1·51	-1·17	29
British whites	1·20	0·16	1·32	-0·76	45	1·55	0·19	1·49	0·30	29
Marital relations										
Happy										
All races	1·46	0·13	1·54	-0·63	115	1·57	0·13	1·72	-1·13	105
British whites	1·42	0·14	1·63	-1·55	89	1·58	0·13	1·75	-1·29	103
Disturbed										
All races	1·41	0·10	1·47	-0·58	170	1·58	0·11	1·56	0·16	142
British whites	1·38	0·10	1·52	-1·41	140	1·54	0·11	1·55	-0·01	125
Frequency of intercourse										
Infrequent (less than 3 times a month)										
All races	1·24	0·16	1·50	-1·59	54	1·97	0·77	1·32	0·86	92
British whites	1·18	0·17	1·49	-1·85	49	1·53	0·14	1·65	-0·82	64
Frequent (3 times a month or more)										
All races	1·55	0·19	1·68	-0·68	29	2·20	1·09	1·15	0·96	64
British whites	1·45	0·20	1·71	-1·35	22	1·65	0·19	1·69	-0·24	37

* Expected means controlled for age at and duration of marriage derived from the Registrar General's Annual Statistical Reviews for England and Wales, Table PP.

Course of Illness

Course of psychosis did not seem to be related to fertility before admission. The schizophrenics and the women suffering from affective disorder showed reduced fertility to an insignificant extent, whether they recovered or not and whether all races or British whites were analysed.

INTERACTION OF SIGNIFICANT VARIABLES IN THE REDUCED FERTILITY BEFORE ADMISSION OF SCHIZOPHRENIC WOMEN

It was decided to cross tabulate the variables of religion, social class, and education for the schizophrenics in order to detect any interaction between these variables. Schizophrenic women whose husbands were classified in social classes I–III were at least 80 per cent Protestant, whereas 52 such women who were married to labourers were only 53·8 per cent Protestant or Jewish, and 46·2 per cent were Roman Catholic; these were probably mainly Irish, or European refugees. In the analysis of schizophrenic women those who were British and white, and were married to manual workers had a more reduced fertility than the fertility of this clinical and sociological group of all races combined. This may be seen as evidence of the interaction discussed. There appeared to be little interaction of religion and education but this was difficult to assess because there were only 22 patients in the sample of ever married schizophrenic women who had received any education after the age of 18. Schizophrenic women who left school at a later age appeared more often to be married to men in non-manual occupations, although the interaction was by no means clear.

It seems likely that the Protestant religion and non-manual occupations are each important variables in producing reduced fertility during the period before admission in spite of the above interactions. It should be emphasized that these fertility differentials were too slight to be sociologically or clinically important, and thus sophisticated analysis of the interaction of such variables was unnecessary.

SUMMARY OF RESULTS ON PRE-PSYCHOTIC FERTILITY

Taking the results based on analysis of British white patients, which permit more reliable comparisons with general population data:

1. Schizophrenic women had on average $1·36 \pm 0·07$ children before their first admission, which was significantly less than the mean family size of $1·54$ expected in the general population, controlled for age at and duration of marriage. However, this difference was too slight to be sociologically important.
2. Women suffering from affective disorders did not differ significantly from the corresponding general population in fertility before admission.
3. Protestant schizophrenic women had a significantly reduced fertility before first admission ($1·33 \pm 0·08$ compared with $1·5$ expected), whereas

Roman Catholic schizophrenic women had a slight but insignificant increase in fertility. Women suffering from affective disorders showed similar differentials by religion to a less significant extent.

4. All social classes of schizophrenic women had some reduction in fertility before admission, but the women suffering from affective disorders who were married to men in non-manual occupations had a statistically significant reduction in fertility ($1 \cdot 45 \pm 0 \cdot 12$ children compared with $1 \cdot 73$ expected).

5. Analysis by the variables of education, marital relations, frequency of sexual intercourse produced little of social importance in either clinical group.

6. There appeared to be some interaction of the variables of religion and social class within the schizophrenics; for example, there was a greater proportion of Roman Catholics among patients married to unskilled labourers. The separate analysis of British white patients probably minimized the effects of this interaction.

CHAPTER XIII

LEGITIMATE FERTILITY AFTER FIRST ADMISSION

INTRODUCTION

THE central aim of the special analysis of fertility after first admission was to assess whether each main clinical group demonstrated a reduction in fertility when controlled comparisons were made with women in the general population. It was considered particularly necessary to evaluate the role of hospitalization in producing any such reduction, in view of the widespread development of community care in Greater London during the years of the follow-up study (1955–66). This evaluation was the most difficult aspect of this survey. As noted in the previous chapter, the basic problem was the difficulty of making adequately controlled comparisons between each main clinical group and women in the general population and between the clinical groups themselves, owing to the disrupting influence of psychosis on marital relations and child-bearing.

An example may illustrate some of the problems involved: first, comparing a patient and a woman from the general population, consider a patient aged 40 who has spent 7 of the past 10 years of her marriage in hospital for treatment of schizophrenia. She was married at 28 and had one child before her first admission at 30, after this she was so paranoid that the marriage was very unhappy. She believed that she was an ambassadress in Britain, that she was being persecuted by Communist agents, and that her husband wished to send her into outer space. Her husband took rigorous precautions against further pregnancies. A woman in the general population, who was married at the same age would probably have had 12 continuous years of married life in which she could have two or more children. It is therefore necessary when comparing the fertility of patients and normal women to pay careful attention to the measurement of special factors influencing the patients, such as hospitalization, course of psychosis, and severe disturbance of marital relations.

Comparisons between two clinical groups present even greater problems. Schizophrenic women tend to be admitted early in their reproductive period, whereas patients with affective disorders are much more likely to become ill at the menopause or later. Suppose the schizophrenic group consisted of one patient married at 20, admitted at 22 and followed-up for 3 further years in which she has two children, and another patient aged 35, married for 15 years with no children, who remains infertile during a year's observation. We need to compare this group with that of two women suffering from affective disorders, one of whom is aged 30 who has just married and has one child during the follow-up, and the other aged 40 married for 20 years with one child, who has another child after her discharge. Both clinical groups have produced two children after discharge, but age differences and differences in marriage duration prevent direct controlled comparison between them. In these circumstances it should be emphasized that the only reliable comparisons made are between each group of patients and normal women, controlled for age at marriage and duration of marriage, as in the analysis of legitimate fertility before first admission.

The method of measuring fertility after admission was as described in detail in CHAPTER VII on data collection and in CHAPTER VIII on statistical methods: further mathematical details are given in Appendix, Part B of the author's Ph.D. thesis. The period after first admission has been measured in two ways: first, from the first admission until the end of the follow-up, so that comparisons with the general population may demonstrate the influence of hospital stay on the fertility of our sample; secondly, the period from the first discharge until the end of the follow-up was taken, in which the expected fertility of the general population was corrected to measure only births conceived during periods when the patients were out of hospital. This method enabled the detection of any reduction in fertility which was independent of the effect of hospitalization (see page 3 of the Questionnaire [page 55] for an example of the latter method).

As in previous analyses, all races were analysed together and then British white patients separately, in order to eliminate a bias towards high fertility by the over-representation of non-British Roman Catholic and coloured patients found in the sample.

GENERAL RESULTS

TABLE 27 gives the general results. Considering the schizophrenic women of all races, they have a statistically significant reduction in fertility after first admission. The 327 schizophrenic patients had a mean family size of 0.39 ± 0.05 compared with 0.53 expected in the general population, but this reduction appeared to depend on the effect of hospitalization, because when this was removed the reduction was no longer statistically significant, i.e. the ratio of actual-expected mean family size to the standard error of the actual mean drops to far less than 2 (-0.93). The British white schizophrenics exhibited a slightly more significantly reduced fertility (a mean family size of 0.37 ± 0.05 compared with 0.52 expected) but this also was largely due to the effect of hospitalization in reducing the period of exposure to the risk of conception. The patients with affective disorders exhibited basically the same trend towards fertility which was mainly dependent on hospitalization, and which is a little more clearly seen when British white patients in this clinical group were analysed, but, unlike the reduction in fertility in the schizophrenics, none of these differences were statistically significant. TABLE 27 demonstrates that when controlled comparisons are made with the general population,

TABLE 27

LEGITIMATE FERTILITY AFTER FIRST ADMISSION OF WOMEN SUFFERING FROM SCHIZOPHRENIA AND AFFECTIVE DISORDERS COMPARED WITH THAT EXPECTED IN THE CORRESPONDING GENERAL POPULATION*: FOR ALL RACES AND BRITISH WHITE PATIENTS ONLY

Ethnic group	Post-psychotic period	Schizophrenics					Affectives				
		Actual mean family size	S.E.	Expected mean	Ratio of actual-expected to S.E.	N	Actual mean family size	S.E.	Expected mean	Ratio of actual-expected to S.E.	N
All races	Post-adm.	0·39	0·05	0·53	–2·96	327	0·33	0·05	0·40	–1·43	262
	Post-dis.†	0·40	0·05	0·44	–0·93	313	0·33	0·05	0·34	–0·28	249
British whites only	Post-adm.	0·37	0·05	0·52	–3·00	265	0·31	0·05	0·39	–1·62	221
	Post-dis.	0·38	0·05	0·43	–1·13	256	0·30	0·05	0·33	–0·74	211

* Expected means, controlled for age at marriage and duration of marriage, derived from the Registrar General's Annual Statistical Reviews for England and Wales, Table PP.
† Expected means controlled for hospitalization in order to detect reductions in fertility independent of periods of in-patient care.

neither clinical group demonstrated a reduction in fertility after discharge large enough to be of any real sociological or eugenic value.

ANALYSIS BY SOCIOLOGICAL VARIABLES: RELIGION AND SOCIAL CLASS

Religion

Analysis by religion and social class [TABLE 28] produced similar differentials to those obtained for the period before first admission. The group of 244 Protestant and Jewish schizophrenic women had a significantly reduced fertility after admission when all races are considered, i.e. reading across this table, they had a mean family size of 0·34±0·05 compared with 0·51 expected. When the 227 British white schizophrenic patients in this religious group were analysed separately the reduction in fertility was slightly more significant, but in both instances the reduction was largely due to the effect of hospital stay in reducing the period of exposure to the risk of conception. The smaller group of 78 Roman Catholic schizophrenics also had a slightly reduced fertility to an insignificant extent, this difference was also dependent upon hospitalization. When the effect of hospital stay was removed they had a statistically insignificant increased fertility when compared with the general population, especially when British white Roman Catholics were analysed separately. However, partly owing to the small size of this religious group and the resultant large standard errors the differentials are nowhere near statistical significance. The patients with affective disorders exhibited basically the same trends as the schizophrenics but to a lesser extent. The reduction in fertility in the Protestant and Jewish women with affective disorders was never significant, whether all races or British white patients were analysed.

Social class as measured by the husbands' occupation produced significant differentials in the fertility after admission of both clinical groups. There was a significant reduction in fertility among 78 schizophrenic women married to non-manual workers which was quite independent of the effect of hospitalization, and this reduction remained when British white patients in this clinical and social category were analysed. For example, 59 British white schizophrenic women married to non-manual workers had a mean family size of 0·29±0·09 compared with 0·50 expected in the general population. The larger group of 195 schizophrenics married to manual workers also had a reduced fertility but this was only significant when the effect of hospital stay was allowed. The analysis of 159 British white women in the latter clinical and social group also showed how the reduction in fertility was dependent upon the effect of hospitalization in the lower social classes. It is interesting that the 65 women of all races suffering from affective disorders who were married to men in non-manual occupations showed a highly significant reduction in fertility after admission whether the period after admission or after discharge was taken, and this reduction remained when only British white patients were

TABLE 28

LEGITIMATE FERTILITY AFTER FIRST ADMISSION OF WOMEN SUFFERING FROM SCHIZOPHRENIA AND AFFECTIVE STATES COMPARED WITH THAT EXPECTED IN NORMAL WOMEN BY RELIGION AND SOCIAL CLASS: FOR ALL RACES AND FOR BRITISH WHITE PATIENTS ONLY

Independent variable	Race	Post-psychotic period*	Schizophrenics					Affectives				
			Actual mean	S.E.	Expected mean	Ratio of actual-expected to S.E.	N	Actual mean	S.E.	Expected mean	Ratio of actual-expected to S.E.	N
Religion												
Protestant and a small group of Jewish patients combined	All	Post-adm.	0·34	0·05	0·51	−3·16	244	0·31	0·05	0·39	−1·53	186
		Post-dis.	0·35	0·05	0·43	−1·54	236	0·30	0·05	0·33	−0·53	175
	British whites	Post-adm.	0·34	0·05	0·52	−3·29	227	0·31	0·05	0·38	−1·22	193
		Post-dis.	0·35	0·06	0·44	−1·72	220	0·30	0·05	0·33	−0·44	184
Roman Catholic	All	Post-adm.	0·46	0·08	0·59	−1·39	78	0·42	0·11	0·43	−0·07	52
		Post-dis.	0·47	0·09	0·47	0·02	72	0·41	0·11	0·37	0·35	51
	British whites	Post-adm.	0·49	0·14	0·53	−0·30	35	0·30	0·13	0·48	−1·48	27
		Post-dis.	0·52	0·15	0·39	0·82	33	0·30	0·13	0·40	0·98	26
Social class												
Non-manual	All	Post-adm.	0·29	0·07	0·53	−3·21	78	0·09	0·04	0·31	−6·06	65
		Post-dis.	0·30	0·07	0·47	−2·25	76	0·10	0·04	0·26	−4·32	62
	British whites	Post-adm.	0·28	0·09	0·57	−3·35	60	0·08	0·03	0·32	−7·33	66
		Post-dis.	0·29	0·09	0·50	−2·43	59	0·08	0·03	0·26	−5·12	62
Manual	All	Post-adm.	0·41	0·06	0·54	−2·14	195	0·37	0·07	0·42	−0·71	124
		Post-dis.	0·41	0·06	0·44	−0·78	187	0·37	0·07	0·36	0·15	117
	British whites	Post-adm.	0·35	0·07	0·53	−2·53	159	0·38	0·08	0·40	−0·22	107
		Post-dis.	0·40	0·07	0·43	−1·03	153	0·38	0·09	0·34	0·46	102

* The 'post-psychotic period' refers to the entire period of the patients' lives after first admission, quite irrespective of whether they recovered, or remained mentally ill.

analysed. For example, in the latter racial group, of 62 women with affective disorders married to non-manual workers, the mean family size was only 0·08 ± 0·3 after discharge compared with 0·26 expected, which is a significant difference, with a high ratio of actual–expected mean to the standard error of the actual mean of − 5·12. The larger group of 124 patients with affective disorders married to manual workers only have an insignificantly reduced fertility after admission which was dependent on the effect of hospital stay. When the period after first discharge was taken those married to manual workers have an insignificantly increased fertility, whether all races or British white patients are analysed.

ANALYSIS BY OTHER SOCIO-PSYCHOLOGICAL VARIABLES: EDUCATION OF PATIENT AND MARITAL RELATIONS

TABLE 29 gives the results of the analysis of fertility after admission by education and the marital relationship. Education did not appear to be a very relevant variable; the schizophrenics again had a significantly reduced fertility which was largely dependent upon the effect of hospital stay, whether all races or British white patients were considered, and this was irrespective of education level. The group of 150 British white schizophrenic women who had received no further education demonstrated a significantly reduced fertility (0·29 ± 0·06 compared with 0·41 expected in the general population) which was independent of the effect of hospitalization. The reasons for this type of reduction is most probably the disturbing effect of the schizophrenic psychosis on the marital relationship, and perhaps caution on the part of the patient's husband to prevent pregnancies which could mean further breakdowns for the patient. The patients with affective disorders did not demonstrate any significant reductions however they were analysed by education.

Schizophrenics, whose husbands or other close relatives emphasized that the marital relationship was happy, had a significantly reduced fertility after admission independent of the effect of hospitalization, this reduction being more apparent in the 86 British white patients in this sub-group [TABLE 29]. However, a larger number of schizophrenics (141) appeared to have disturbed marriages and the significant reduction in their fertility depended upon the effect of hospitalization. It should be emphasized that these results are only based on those case notes giving details of marital relations, and therefore no clear statement can be made as to the proportions experiencing disturbed but unbroken marriages. It seems possible that the more happily married couples adjusted to the problems associated with the patient's illness and limited their families in order to avoid further breakdowns, whereas those with disturbed relations were in hospital longer and their fertility was more diminished by this separation from their husbands.

Considering the women suffering from affective disorders, there appeared to be a much lower proportion of disturbed marriages than was found among the schizophrenics. The only significant reduction in fertility of the group of

TABLE 29

LEGITIMATE FERTILITY AFTER FIRST ADMISSION OF WOMEN SUFFERING FROM SCHIZOPHRENIA AND AFFECTIVE STATES COMPARED WITH THAT EXPECTED IN NORMAL WOMEN, BY EDUCATION AND MARITAL RELATIONS: FOR ALL RACES AND BRITISH WHITE PATIENTS ONLY

Independent variable	Race	Post-psychotic period	Schizophrenics					Affectives				
			Actual mean	S.E.	Expected mean	Ratio of actual-expected to S.E.	N	Actual mean	S.E.	Expected mean	Ratio of actual-expected to S.E.	N
No further education	All	Post-adm.	0·33	0·05	0·51	-3·42	186	0·34	0·06	0·39	-0·77	173
		Post-dis.	0·34	0·05	0·43	-1·57	176	0·32	0·06	0·32	-0·01	164
	British whites	Post-adm.	0·29	0·05	0·50	-3·86	157	0·32	0·06	0·38	-0·83	157
		Post-dis.	0·29	0·06	0·41	-2·03	150	0·31	0·06	0·33	-0·30	150
Some further education	All	Post-adm.	0·38	0·09	0·63	-2·57	60	0·25	0·17	0·30	-0·32	16
		Post-dis.	0·39	0·11	0·55	-1·52	56	0·27	0·18	0·21	0·30	15
	British whites	Post-adm.	0·35	0·11	0·69	-3·05	43	0·24	0·13	0·29	-0·36	21
		Post-dis.	0·37	0·12	0·60	-1·96	41	0·25	0·14	0·22	0·23	20
Marital relations												
Happy	All	Post-adm.	0·28	0·06	0·47	-3·24	105	0·27	0·07	0·37	-1·35	88
		Post-dis.	0·28	0·06	0·41	-2·20	103	0·27	0·08	0·31	-0·51	84
	British whites	Post-adm.	0·26	0·06	0·48	-3·33	87	0·23	0·07	0·34	-1·53	86
		Post-dis.	0·27	0·06	0·42	-2·41	86	0·24	0·07	0·30	-0·88	84
Disturbed	All	Post-adm.	0·33	0·07	0·56	-3·25	141	0·28	0·07	0·43	-2·21	75
		Post-dis.	0·33	0·08	0·44	-1·43	131	0·27	0·07	0·38	-1·44	73
	British whites	Post-adm.	0·32	0·08	0·55	-2·69	118	0·40	0·09	0·47	-0·77	68
		Post-dis.	0·33	0·09	0·43	-1·07	111	0·40	0·09	0·41	-0·06	65

women suffering from affective disorders, when analysed by this variable, was among 75 patients of all races whose marriages were disturbed; even this significant reduction was dependent upon the effect of hospitalization. The more reliable analysis of women suffering from affective disorders who were British and white indicated that any reduction in their fertility after admission was statistically and sociologically insignificant. However, owing to the lack of adequate data on marital relations in many case notes too much reliability cannot be attached to this aspect of the analysis. A more intensive inquiry involving interviews to evaluate marital relations is definitely necessary for more reliable findings.

ANALYSIS BY OTHER CLINICAL VARIABLES

Analysis by length of hospital stay has produced some results which are difficult to interpret. TABLE 30 indicates that the proportion of women in both clinical groups who experienced a total length of hospital stay of under one year was greater than the proportion staying in hospital for longer periods. This demonstrated the trend towards short periods of in-patient care and the development of community care for the mentally ill in Greater London during the period of the survey (1955–66). It should be remembered that the method of sampling excluded the group of very long-stay institutionalized schizo-phrenics whose fertility was assessed in a pilot study [see CHAPTER IV]. The 152 schizophrenic women who were British and white and whose total length of hospital stay was under one year had a clearly reduced fertility quite indepen-dent of the effect of hospitalization. However, patients with this diagnosis who were in hospital for longer periods did not show a statistically significant reduction in fertility after admission when only those among them who were British and white were analysed. This surprising result may be due to the smaller size of the long-stay British white group (89) and resultant large standard errors, so that significant differences were more difficult to detect. The analysis suggested that a larger sample of long-stay schizophrenic women would demonstrate significantly reduced fertility after admission but that this reduction would be mainly the result of hospitalization. The reduced fertility of the long-stay patients appeared to be more dependent on in-patient care than the reduced fertility of short-stay patients as would be expected, i.e. the more hospitalization the greater its effect. The women with affective disorders showed some reductions: all those 180 patients who were only in hospital a short time did not have a significantly reduced fertility. The small group of 28 British white women staying longer in hospital for treatment of an affective illness had a highly significant reduction, which was clearly independent of the basic effect of hospitalization in reducing exposure to conception. How-ever, women with affective disorders who stay in hospital for long periods are a small atypical group and in no way representative of the entire sample of women suffering from these illnesses, so that caution is necessary in interpret-ing these particular estimates.

TABLE 30

LEGITIMATE FERTILITY AFTER ADMISSION OF WOMEN SUFFERING FROM SCHIZOPHRENIA AND AFFECTIVE DISORDERS COMPARED WITH THAT EXPECTED IN NORMAL WOMEN BY LENGTH OF HOSPITALIZATION: FOR ALL RACES AND BRITISH WHITE PATIENTS SEPARATELY

Independent variable	Race	Post-psychotic period	Schizophrenics					Affectives				
			Actual mean	S.E.	Expected mean	Ratio of actual-expected to S.E.	N	Actual mean	S.E.	Expected mean	Ratio of actual-expected to S.E.	N
Hospitalization up to last discharge from hospital chosen	All	Post-adm.	0·34	0·05	0·44	-1·90	201	0·29	0·05	0·32	-0·48	180
		Post-dis.	0·35	0·05	0·41	-1·16	199	0·29	0·06	0·30	-0·06	178
	British whites	Post-adm.	0·26	0·05	0·43	-3·16	152	0·29	0·06	0·32	-0·64	171
		Post-dis.	0·26	0·05	0·39	-2·51	151	0·29	0·06	0·30	-0·17	168
Under 1 year	All	Post-adm.	0·45	0·10	0·64	-1·91	101	0·28	0·11	0·61	-3·00	32
		Post-dis.	0·45	0·10	0·48	-0·28	99	0·28	0·11	0·50	-1·99	32
	British whites	Post-adm.	0·44	0·11	0·63	-1·79	89	0·07	0·05	0·60	-10·81	28
		Post-dis.	0·45	0·11	0·48	-0·31	87	0·07	0·05	0·48	-8·37	28
1-10 + years	All	Post-adm.	0·43	0·12	0·47	-1·16	30	0·31	0·17	0·25	0·35	13
		Post-dis.	0·32	0·12	0·41	-0·69	28	0·31	0·17	0·22	0·51	13
	British whites	Post-adm.	0·14	0·08	0·42	-3·57	21	0·31	0·17	0·27	0·23	13
		Post-dis.	0·15	0·08	0·38	-2·88	20	0·31	0·17	0·27	0·41	13
Hospitalization in follow-up												
Under 1 year	All	Post-adm.	0·67	0·25	0·57	0·40	12	0·00	0·57	0·32	-0·57	1
		Post-dis.	0·58	0·22	0·35	1·07	12	0·00	0·51	0·26	-0·51	1
1-10 + years	British whites	Post-adm.	0·60	0·25	0·49	0·45	10	0·00	0·57	0·32	-0·57	1
		Post-dis.	0·60	0·25	0·32	1·09	10	0·00	0·51	0·26	-0·51	1

FURTHER ANALYSIS BY FREQUENCY OF INTERCOURSE AND COURSE OF PSYCHOSIS

TABLE 31 gives the results of analysis by frequency of intercourse and course of psychosis for those patients whose case notes gave adequate information. Schizophrenic women having intercourse less than three times a month had a significantly reduced fertility independent of the effect of hospitalization and irrespective of racial origin, whereas those having more frequent intercourse showed no such significant reduction. The women suffering from affective disorders did not have a reduced fertility to any significant extent but demonstrated the trend towards less fertility, especially among those having infrequent intercourse, whether all patients or British white patients were analysed. However, as in the case when marital relations were considered, there were inadequate data on frequency of intercourse in most of the case notes so that little reliability may be attached to this particular aspect of the analysis.

In respect of the course of psychosis up to the end of the follow-up, the larger group of schizophrenics who definitely did not recover had a significantly reduced fertility regardless of race but this obviously depended upon the effect of hospitalization. Among those schizophrenic women who recovered, the reduction in fertility was not statistically significant however analysed. Again, women suffering from affective disorders did not appear to differ significantly from the general population but those patients of this diagnosis who did not recover showed a tendency towards reduced fertility, which was more detectable in the British white patients; those women suffering from affective disorders who recovered showed an insignificantly increased fertility, which was more apparent in the analysis of all races than in the separate analysis of those patients who were British and white.

THERAPEUTIC ABORTIONS AND STERILIZATIONS

Fertility after first admission was also analysed separately for those patients who did not receive therapeutic abortions or sterilization, compared with those few who did. There were 240 British white schizophrenics who did not receive any such gynaecological treatment and their fertility was significantly reduced after admission, but this was largely dependent upon the effect of hospital stay. Out of the 20 schizophrenics who had abortions or sterilization only the 15 British white patients showed a significant reduction in fertility which was not dependent upon the effect of hospitalization. The 210 British white women suffering from affective disorders who received no therapeutic abortions or sterilizations had a reduced fertility, but as is usual in this group of patients this difference was insignificant whether or not the effect of hospital stay was allowed for and when all races of patients were analysed together. The very small group of 11 women suffering from affective disorders who had therapeutic abortions or sterilizations showed a significantly reduced fertility

TABLE 31

LEGITIMATE FERTILITY AFTER FIRST ADMISSION OF WOMEN SUFFERING FROM SCHIZOPHRENIA AND AFFECTIVE STATES COMPARED WITH THAT EXPECTED IN CORRESPONDING NORMAL WOMEN BY FREQUENCY OF SEXUAL INTERCOURSE AND COURSE OF PSYCHOSIS: FOR ALL RACES AND BRITISH WHITES SEPARATELY

Independent variable	Race	Post-psychotic period	Schizophrenics					Affectives				
			Actual mean	S.E.	Expected mean	Ratio of actual-expected to S.E.	N	Actual mean	S.E.	Expected mean	Ratio of actual-expected to S.E.	N
Frequency of intercourse												
Infrequent (less than 3 times monthly)	All	Post-adm.	0·22	0·07	0·50	−4·11	54	0·16	0·05	0·25	−1·69	73
		Post-dis.	0·24	0·07	0·39	−2·02	50	0·14	0·05	0·18	−0·69	71
	British whites	Post-adm.	0·17	0·07	0·51	−4·83	47	0·28	0·08	0·38	−1·38	47
		Post-dis.	0·19	0·08	0·38	−2·61	43	0·24	0·08	0·27	−0·37	45
Frequent (3 times a month or more)	All	Post-adm.	0·35	0·13	0·46	−0·85	23	0·22	0·09	0·28	−0·70	55
		Post-dis.	0·38	0·14	0·39	−0·09	21	0·22	0·09	0·24	−0·20	54
	British whites	Post-adm.	0·35	0·15	0·47	−0·81	20	0·33	0·15	0·42	−0·55	30
		Post-dis.	0·37	0·15	0·37	−0·12	19	0·33	0·15	0·34	−0·07	30
Course of psychosis												
Not recovered	All	Post-adm.	0·39	0·07	0·57	−2·64	122	0·28	0·07	0·37	−1·23	95
		Post-dis.	0·39	0·07	0·46	−0·98	120	0·29	0·07	0·29	−0·11	91
	British whites	Post-adm.	0·34	0·07	0·55	−3·10	95	0·28	0·07	0·37	−1·25	83
		Post-dis.	0·34	0·07	0·44	1·38	94	0·28	0·08	0·30	−0·28	80
Recovered	All	Post-adm.	0·30	0·09	0·42	−1·35	76	0·45	0·13	0·31	1·10	58
		Post-dis.	0·31	0·09	0·39	−0·95	75	0·46	0·13	0·28	1·43	56
	British whites	Post-adm.	0·30	0·09	0·40	−1·11	67	0·40	0·13	0·34	0·52	52
		Post-dis.	0·30	0·10	0·38	−0·78	66	0·42	0·13	0·31	0·84	50

when all races were analysed together, but this depended on hospital stay. The six British white women in this clinical group having abortions or sterilizations showed no significant reduction in fertility. It should be emphasized that the proportion of each clinical group who received such treatment is too small to be socially important, and there seemed to be little effect of such therapy on the total fertility of these groups after admission. A larger sample of patients receiving such gynaecological treatment would be necessary in order to relate time of operation to course of illness in assessing fertility differentials.

It should be emphasized that since probability of marriage is higher before illness than afterwards, most of the fertility after admission discussed above is the fertility of marriages which were contracted before the patient's first admission. A separate analysis of the small group of patients of all races who married after first discharge indicated a somewhat different pattern: 43 schizophrenics who married during this period had a mean family size of $1 \cdot 07 \pm 0 \cdot 22$ compared with $1 \cdot 21$ expected in the general population, but this reduced fertility was not significant and it depended entirely on the effect of hospitalization. Thus the schizophrenic women who married after their first admission did not appear to exhibit the statistically significant reduction in fertility which was found in the analysis of the fertility after admission of marriages contracted before first admission. The women suffering from affective disorders showed the opposite trend: whereas their fertility after admission as a whole was not significantly reduced when compared with the general population; the small group of 11 women suffering from affective disorders who contracted a marriage after first admission and gave adequate information, had a statistically significantly reduced fertility independent of the effect of hospitalization. However, the small size of this group and their differential fertility are of little clinical or sociological importance.

INTERACTION OF VARIABLES IN THE POST-PSYCHOTIC FERTILITY OF SCHIZOPHRENICS

In the above analysis the size of the sample allowed the rigorous control of age at marriage, duration of marriage and hospitalization, in the comparison of specific sociological groups within each clinical category with women in the general population. However, it was not possible to undertake a more multi-factorial approach because this would have resulted in too small numbers in each cell for the reliable estimation of fertility differentials. Since only the schizophrenics demonstrated a persistent reduction in fertility after admission, which was statistically significant, it was decided to limit the study of the interaction of variables to this clinical group.

Cross tabulations of the variables of social class, hospital stay, marital relations, and course of psychosis showed some interaction between them.

First, considering social class and hospital stay, there were fewer patients married to non-manual workers in the long-stay groups. For example, among 32 schizophrenics who were in hospital for under one month $28 \cdot 3$ per cent were married to non-manual workers compared with only 10·8 per cent of patients staying in hospital for 2–5 years. This interaction may partially explain why the reduction in fertility of the non-manual group was independent of the effect of hospitalization, i.e. fewer of this group were long-stay cases compared with those in the manual group, where the effect of hospitalization on fertility was more apparent [TABLE 28].

Social class also seemed to interact with marital relations. More women with happy marriages were married to non-manual workers than the women with disturbed marriages found in this social category. However, these differences were not large and in view of the nature of the information involved too much reliability cannot be attached to them. Cross tabulation of marital relations by length of stay demonstrated a tendency for those with happy marriages to be short-stay cases; only 26·1 per cent of happily married patients stayed in hospital for more than one year compared with 33·2 per cent of the patients having more disturbed marital relations. Some association between happy marriages, short stays in hospital, and marriage to non-manual workers seems probable, and this would account for the reduced fertility of those with happy marriages which is independent of the effect of hospitalization [TABLE 29]. Marital relations and course of psychosis appeared to interact: 44·3 per cent of recovered schizophrenic women had happy marriages compared with 31 per cent of schizophrenic women who were in hospital at the time of follow-up. Social class bears some relationship to course of psychosis; only 46·7 per cent of the schizophrenic patients who appeared to recover were married to manual workers compared with 74·1 per cent in this social class among those in hospital at the follow-up.

Neither religion nor education appeared to interact significantly with length of stay. In view of the lack of sociologically important findings on fertility after admission, more sophisticated analysis of the interaction of variables appears unprofitable.

SUMMARY OF RESULTS ON FERTILITY AFTER FIRST ADMISSION

Taking the results on British white patients, which permit the most reliable comparisons with the general population of women:

1. After admission, the fertility of schizophrenic women was significantly reduced, i.e. 265 such patients had a mean family size of 0·37±0·05 children compared with 0·52 expected; this reduction was largely dependent on the effect of hospitalization in reducing exposure to risk of conception. Although the reduction is statistically significant, it is not large enough to be of any real clinical, sociological, or eugenic importance.

    The women with affective disorders did not demonstrate a statistically significant reduction in fertility after admission.

2. Protestant schizophrenic women had a significantly reduced fertility, but

Roman Catholic schizophrenics and all religious groups of women suffering from affective disorders did not differ significantly from the general population.

3. Women married to non-manual workers in both clinical groups had a significantly reduced fertility, which was independent of the effect of hospitalization; the groups of schizophrenics with husbands in manual occupations had a reduced fertility, the statistical significance of which depended upon the effect of hospital stay.

4. Among the schizophrenics, those who were happily married and those who had no further education had a reduced fertility independent of hospitalization, whereas those whose marriages were unhappy and those having further education only had a reduction in fertility which was dependent on the effect of hospitalization.

5. Short-stay schizophrenics had a reduced fertility independent of hospitalization, but the reduction in long-stay cases was not quite statistically significant, probably because of the smaller size of the long-stay sample rendering differentials more difficult to assess. A small atypical group of long-stay affectives had a significantly reduced fertility.

6. Schizophrenics who had infrequent intercourse had a significantly reduced fertility not accounted for by hospitalization, whereas the smaller group whose notes gave evidence that intercourse was more frequent showed no decreased fertility. Women suffering from affective disorders showed a similar trend to an insignificant extent. Too much reliability cannot be given to these particular findings because most case records gave inadequate data on this variable.

7. Schizophrenics who recovered had no significant fertility differentials but those who did not had a significantly reduced fertility which was obviously dependent upon the effect of hospitalization in reducing the periods of exposure to the risk of conception.

8. Preliminary analysis of the interaction of variables suggested some association between husbands in non-manual occupations, happy marriages, and short stay in hospital among the schizophrenics.

9. Analysis by all these variables clearly demonstrated that during recent years of developing community care of the mentally ill, none of the statistically significant reductions in the fertility of our sample after admission are large enough to be clinically or sociologically important, or of any eugenic value. The relevance of this finding in relation to those of studies before the advent of community-orientated psychiatry is discussed in CHAPTER XVIII.

CHAPTER XIV

CHANGES IN MARITAL STATUS: SEPARATION AND DIVORCE

INTRODUCTION

DATA on marital status changes appeared complex, and in order to present a clear analysis information was coded separately for changes during the following three periods of the patients' lives: (1) the period before first admission; (2) the period between first admission and last discharge; and (3) the period from last discharge from the hospital selected until the end of observation.

Each patient was allowed on the coding scheme three possible changes in marital status during each of these periods; the results indicated that only a very small group of patients of each diagnosis experienced more than one change during each period. As in the special analysis of marriage and fertility [CHAPTERS X to XIII] the group of patients known to be suffering from serious physical illness associated with their mental state were excluded from this analysis of changes in marital status.

MARITAL STATUS CHANGES BEFORE FIRST ADMISSION

TABLE 32 gives the percentage distribution of marital status changes by diagnosis for the period before admission for first marriages only. More of the women suffering from affective disorders had married, not only because they were older than the schizophrenics on first admission but because of their higher probability of marriage before admission [CHAPTER X], and therefore more of them are exposed to the risk of separation or divorce during this period. If the proportion of ever married who became separated or divorced is calculated as an index of marital disruption, 17·9 per cent of 407 schizophrenics and 15·7 per cent of 388 women suffering from affective disorders parted from their first husbands. The difference between these proportions is insignificant statistically. Patients who experienced a temporary separation but who were eventually reconciled with their husbands are not included in these proportions. Ten schizophrenic women married for a second time and three of these marriages were ended by separation or divorce before first admission; 18 women suffering from affective disorders had second marriages, three of which ended in separation during this period. Only one patient, a schizophrenic, had been married three times and all of her marriages had failed.

CHANGES IN MARITAL STATUS AFTER FIRST ADMISSION

TABLES 33 and 34 show marital status changes by diagnosis for the period after first admission, TABLE 33 for the period from admission until last

TABLE 32

PERCENTAGE DISTRIBUTION OF MARITAL STATUS CHANGES BEFORE FIRST ADMISSION BY DIAGNOSIS

| Diagnosis | First ever marital status change | | | | | | | | | N |
	None	Married for 1st time	Separated	Separated and reconciled	Divorced	Marriage declared null	Widowed	Reconciled and widowed	N.K.	
Schizophrenia	55·3	35·6	3·8	0·2	3·2	0·4	1·1	–	0·4	533
Paranoid schizophrenia	34·9	43·6	9·3	–	7·6	–	4·1	–	0·6	172
Catatonic schizophrenia	53·8	35·9	2·6	–	2·6	–	5·1	–	–	39
Schizo-affectives	43·5	49·3	1·4	–	2·9	–	2·9	–	–	69
Affective disorders	19·5	64·5	6·6	–	6·0	–	2·9	0·2	0·2	482
Total—all diagnoses	38·6	48·2	5·4	0·1	4·8	0·2	2·4	0·1	0·3	1,295

TABLE 33

PERCENTAGE DISTRIBUTION OF MARITAL STATUS CHANGES BETWEEN FIRST EVER ADMISSION AND LAST DISCHARGE BY DIAGNOSIS

Diagnosis	N.A.*	None	Married	Separated	Separated and reconciled	Divorced	Marriage declared null	Div. on grds of insanity	Widowed	N.K.	N
Schizophrenia	25·9	59·1	5·8	4·1	0·9	2·1	0·4	0·2	0·8	0·8	533
Paranoid schizophrenia	40·1	49·4	2·3	2·3	1·2	1·7	–	–	1·2	1·7	172
Catatonic schizophrenia	33·3	59·0	2·6	–	2·6	–	–	–	–	2·6	39
Schizo-affectives	29·0	59·4	5·8	4·3	–	–	–	–	1·4	–	69
Affective disorders	48·5	42·5	2·1	2·1	0·4	–	–	–	1·5	0·4	482
Total—all diagnoses	36·6	51·7	3·9	3·0	0·8	0·2	0·2	0·1	1·1	0·8	1,295

* N.A. = Not applicable, i.e. no period after admission.

TABLE 34

PERCENTAGE DISTRIBUTION OF MARITAL STATUS CHANGES DURING THE FOLLOW-UP BY DIAGNOSIS

Diagnosis	N.A.*	None	Married	Separated	Separated and Reconciled	Divorced	Marriage declared null	Div. on grds of insanity	Widowed	Reconciled and widowed	N.K.	N
Schizophrenia	15·2	55·2	3·2	1·9	0·8	2·1	0·4	0·2	0·4	–	20·8	533
Paranoid schizophrenia	10·5	58·1	1·2	3·5	0·6	4·1	–	–	1·2	–	20·9	172
Catatonic schizophrenia	15·4	59·0	–	2·6	–	2·6	–	–	–	–	20·5	39
Schizo-affectives	10·1	63·8	5·8	1·4	1·4	–	–	–	–	–	17·4	69
Affective disorders	3·5	63·5	3·1	1·2	–	2·7	0·2	–	1·7	0·2	23·9	482
Total—all diagnoses	10·0	59·2	2·9	1·9	0·5	2·5	0·2	0·1	0·9	0·1	21·8	1295

*N.A. = Not applicable, i.e. no period after admission.

discharge, and TABLE 34 for the period from last discharge until the end of the follow-up. Although the largest group of patients of each diagnosis are those experiencing no change in marital status, 18·3 per cent of 470 ever married schizophrenic women became separated or divorced during the period after admission compared with only 10·2 per cent of 413 women suffering from affective disorders. *The difference between these proportions is statistically significant at the one per cent level.* All statistical tests are given in Appendix 5 of the author's Ph.D. thesis. Two schizophrenics and three affectives also parted from their second husband during this period. These estimates include marriages contracted before and after admission.

It was not possible to add together the percentage separated and divorced before and after illness because a few patients who were separated on first admission may have become divorced during subsequent observation. However, even taking the estimates before and after admission separately, both schizophrenics and women suffering from affective disorders seemed especially prone to separation and divorce when compared with women in the general population. Rowntree (1964) gives the proportion of marriages of 10–20 years' duration ending in separation or divorce in England and Wales as between 6·5 and 10·2 per cent; these estimates were based partly on war-time marriages. *The patients of both diagnoses exceed this proportion before illness and the schizophrenics afterwards. It would appear that the crucial factor in marital disruption of these patients is their personality rather than their psychosis and its more immediate problems.*

ANALYSIS OF SEPARATION AND DIVORCE BY THE RELEVANT SOCIOLOGICAL VARIABLES

Analysis was attempted of frequency of separation and divorce in the sample by duration of marriage, age of marriage, religion, occupation of husband, family size, personality, age on first admission, length of hospital stay, and marital relations. The small group of marriages contracted after admission was not included in this particular aspect of the analysis.

Duration of Marriage

TABLE 35 shows that more marriages appeared to have ended within their first 10 years than in their second 10 years. This was mainly due to the fact that the period of observation ended in 1966, and therefore in respect of those patients who married in 1950 or later complete information was not available about separation and divorce during the second 10 years of marriage. If marriages of 1944 or earlier were considered, the number of marriages broken by divorce or separation at durations under 10 years is almost the same as those broken at durations 10–19 years. TABLE 35 combines all ended marriages, whether ended by divorce, separation, or widowhood. Rowntree's (1964) estimates for normal women of corresponding marriage date are given in TABLE 36.

TABLE 35

DURATION OF ENDED MARRIAGES BY DATE OF MARRIAGE IN RELATION TO ALL MARRIAGES: SCHIZOPHRENICS COMPARED WITH AFFECTIVES*

Quinquennial date of marriage	Schizophrenics					Affectives				
	Duration of ended marriages			No. of marriages not ended	Ended marriages as a percentage of all marriages	Duration of ended marriages			No. of marriages not ended	Ended marriages as a percentage of all marriages
	Under 10 yrs	10–19 years	Over 20 yrs			Under 10 yrs	10–19 years	Over 20 yrs		
1925–9	2	1	–	2	60·0	–	–	–	1	–
1930–4	3	2	4	17	34·6	2	3	1	28	17·6
1935–9	5	8	4	41	29·3	6	8	6	60	25·0
1940–4	11	9	–	42	32·2	9	8	–	37	31·5
1945–9	18	13	–	69	31·0	12	6	–	60	23·1
1950–4	11	–	–	52	17·5	11	–	–	42	20·8
1955–9	9	–	–	34	20·9	6	–	–	41	12·8
1960s	1	–	–	16	5·9	3	–	–	10	23·1
N.K.	–	–	–	26	–	1	–	–	23	4·2
Total	60	33	8	299	25·3	50	25	7	302	21·3

* 1955–63 admission sample followed-up until August 1966.

TABLE 36

PERCENTAGE OF MARRIAGES ENDING IN ANY FORM OF SEPARATION OR
WIDOWHOOD BY DATE OF MARRIAGE: ROWNTREE'S SAMPLE FROM THE
GENERAL POPULATION*

Date of marriage	Total N	Percentage ending in separation or divorce	Percentage ending in widowhood	Total ended marriages as percentage of all marriages
1930–4	274	6·5	8·0	14·5
1935–9	361	9·1	7·5	16·6
1940–4	322	10·2	6·5	16·7
1945–9	383	7·8	1·6	9·4

*SOURCE: Rowntree, G. (1964) *Pop. Studies*, Vol. XVIII, No. 2, p. 147. Date of collection of data—1959–60.

The percentage of our patients whose marriages have ended [TABLE 35] is therefore greater than would be expected on the basis of the general population, especially in view of the fact that all Rowntree's marriages were 10–20 years' duration, whereas at least 15 per cent of the patients in each clinical group has marriages of under 10 years' duration. The high percentage of patients parting from their husbands [TABLES 32–35] accounts for the excess of ended marriages in the sample rather than an excess of widowed patients.

The proportion of patients who were widowed on first admission was similar when the two main clinical groups are compared: 4·3 per cent of the schizophrenics and 3·9 per cent of the women suffering from affective disorders had lost their first husbands. After admission slightly more women with affective disorders were known to have been widowed, 4·0 per cent compared with only 2·3 per cent of the schizophrenics. This difference is probably due to two factors: first, that the women with affective disorders were an older group whose husbands were slightly more likely to die than the younger husbands of the schizophrenics, and secondly, that the wife's affective disorder was sometimes reactive to serious physical illness in the husband, who may subsequently have died after her admission.

Age of Patient at First Marriage

During the period before admission in both clinical groups the proportion of patients parting from their husbands was highest when the patient was under 20 at marriage. This agrees with Rowntree's results (1964) based on the general population, although exact comparisons are difficult owing to variations in marriage duration between her sample and ours. Analysis of the period after admission produced no such clear differences in proportions parting by age at marriage in either clinical group.

Religion

Analysis of first marriages of schizophrenics during the period before admission indicated that there were no differences in proportion parting from their husbands by religion (15·9 per cent of the Protestants parted and 15·7 per cent of the Roman Catholics). However, among the women suffering from affective illnesses 12·9 per cent of the Protestants and 21 per cent of the Roman Catholics parted from their husbands, which agrees with Rowntree's finding that more of the Roman Catholics parted (11·7 per cent of the Roman Catholics compared with 7·8 per cent of the Protestants). This finding appeared surprising in view of the Roman Catholic doctrines against divorce; it is probable that many people who give their faith as Roman Catholic do not adhere strictly to the doctrines involved. In our sample, patients of both religions show a greater frequency of marital breakdown than women in the general population. Data on religion of husband were not obtained, and in view of this and differences between clinical groups in duration of marriage, no analysis was undertaken of proportions parting after admission by religion.

Occupation of Husband

The results on the proportion who parted from their husband were difficult to analyse by this variable, because on each main clinical group a large proportion of patients had given no information on husbands' occupation. As would perhaps be expected, it was among the latter group that the proportion who had parted was especially high.

First, considering the 400 schizophrenic women who were married before admission, 20·3 per cent of 94 of those who were married to men in non-manual occupations had become separated or divorced during the period before admission, compared with only 7·9 per cent of 214 such women married to men in manual occupations. This difference in proportions by social class is greater than that found by Rowntree (1964), whose results were based on a random sample of women in the general population of England and Wales. She discovered that during the past 30 years only 9·2 per cent of 392 women married to non-manual workers had become separated or divorced, compared with 7·3 per cent of 466 women married to skilled manual workers, and 9·1 per cent of 465 women married to unskilled manual workers. However, it should be remembered that 92 of the 300 schizophrenic women gave no information regarding their husband's occupation, and in this particular subgroup 39 per cent had parted from their husbands.

The 384 women suffering from affective disorders did not show such clear differences in proportions parting by occupation of husband as those found among the schizophrenics before admission. Out of 97 women with affective illnesses who were married to non-manual workers 7·2 per cent had parted before admission, compared with 9·5 per cent of 179 such women married to men in non-manual occupations. Although these proportions are nearer Rowntree's estimates, it should be emphasized that there were 108 women in this clinical group whose notes contained no information about occupation, and among these 34 per cent had parted from their husbands.

After admission, the difference between proportions parting by occupation among schizophrenic women was not so great, and in fact appeared to be the opposite trend to that found before admission in this clinical group: 15·7 per cent of 159 such women who were married to manual workers had parted compared with only 10·2 per cent of 59 women married to men in non-manual occupations, during this period between first admission and last discharge from the hospital studied. However, out of 59 schizophrenic women giving no information on their husbands' occupation, 22 per cent parted from their husbands during this period.

Among the group of women suffering from affective disorders 12·2 per cent of the 49 in the non-manual category parted from their husbands during the period between first admission and last discharge, compared with only 3·2 per cent of 95 such patients married to men in manual occupations. Again, of 49 such women who gave no information on their husbands' occupation, 22 per cent had parted during this period, between first admission and last discharge from hospital. Unfortunately, in view of the lack of information on husband's occupation among these patients who had become separated or divorced, little reliability can be attached to these particular results.

Family Size

Before admission, separation and divorce were more frequent among patients of both diagnoses who had had fewer than two children. After admission the relationship between proportions parting from their husbands and number of births after admission was not clear owing to the small number of patients bearing children during this period. The results tend to agree with Rowntree's (1964), but our patients are more prone to marital disruption than normal women, irrespective of family size.

Personality

The relationship between pre-morbid personality and marital disruption was difficult to detect owing to the small size of the groups [TABLE 37]. However, during the period before first admission patients of hitherto normal disposition seemed less likely to part from their husbands than those of pronounced abnormal traits in both clinical groups (although the atypical schizoid affectives demonstrated a very low proportion parting which was possibly due to the small numbers in this sub-group. When the test for the significance of the difference between proportions parting was applied to the schizophrenic group, the differences between the abnormal and normal personality groups did not quite reach significance at the 5 per cent level [TABLE 37]. No analysis was undertaken of the marital status changes after admission by personality in view of the small size of the sub-groups of personality, lessened even further by the 20 per cent non-response rate.

Age on First Admission

As one would expect, during the period before admission the proportion of

TABLE 37

NUMBER OF MARRIED PATIENTS PARTING FROM THEIR HUSBANDS BEFORE FIRST ADMISSION BY PRE-MORBID PERSONALITY AND DIAGNOSIS

	Schizophrenics			Affectives		
Personality	*N*	*No. separated or divorced*	*Percentage parting**	*N*	*No. separated or divorced*	*Percentage parting*
1. Schizoid or paranoid	64	13	20·0	45	2	4·4
2. Subject to variable moods	49	13 ⎫		42	9 ⎫	
3. Neurotic traits	39	2 ⎬ 19·8		64	8 ⎬ 18·0	
4. Combination of first three	33	9 ⎭		33	8 ⎭	
5. Impossible to code (includes psychopathic personalities)	50	8	16·0	53	10	18·9
6. Normal	85	10	11·8	95	13	13·7
Not known	87	19	21·8	56	11	19·6
Total	407	74		388	61	

* The differences between proportion of schizophrenics parting in categories 1–4 (abnormal), and category 6 (normal) was not quite significant at the 5 per cent level.

schizophrenics who parted from their husbands increased with age on first admission. However, women suffering from affective disorders showed no such clear relationship between the length of the period before first admission and such severe marital disruption. After admission, in both clinical groups most separations and divorces appeared to occur to patients who were admitted between the ages of 20 and 40 rather than to the very young or middle-aged patients.

Length of Stay

TABLE 38 shows how the proportion of patients who parted from their husbands during the period after admission appeared to increase as length of

TABLE 38

PROPORTION OF PATIENTS PARTING FROM THEIR HUSBANDS DURING THE PERIOD AFTER ADMISSION BY DIAGNOSIS AND LENGTH OF HOSPITAL STAY

Total length of stay	N	Schizophrenics Percentage separated or divorced	N	Affectives Percentage separated or divorced
Under 6 months	82	6·1[a]	79	5·1
6 months to 2 years	107	16·8[b]	67	9·0
Over 2 years	64	25·0[a]	16	18·8

[a] The difference in proportion parting between the very short-stay and long-stay schizophrenics was significant at the 1 per cent level.

[b] The actual difference between the very short-stay and the medium-stay schizophrenics was significant at the 5 per cent level.

hospital stay increased in both clinical groups. *The difference between the proportion of schizophrenics who parted from their husbands was significant at the one per cent level when the very short-stay group was compared with the long-stay group* [TABLE 38, footnote a]. The group of schizophrenics whose total length of hospital stay was of medium duration also parted from the husbands more frequently than the very short-stay group, this difference being only just significant at the 5 per cent level. No such differences were statistically significant among the women suffering from affective disorders, partly because of the small size of the long-stay group of this diagnosis.

Marital Relations

An attempt was made to examine the causes of marital disharmony among those patients who had parted from their husbands during the period between first admission and last discharge (data on such intimate problems was not collected in the postal follow-up). About one-third of each clinical group described their marriage as happy at the time of first admission; among patients' records giving sufficient information the illness itself did not appear to be the main cause of marital breakdown; extra-marital affairs of the husband or patient seemed of equal importance. Significantly more schizophrenics than women suffering from affective disorders parted during this period, perhaps partly because of the age factor, i.e. the former clinical group were younger and their marriages had had less chance to become stable than those of the women suffering from affective illnesses. An interesting finding was that 19 per cent of the marriages of patients in the latter clinical groups were described as never having been satisfactory compared with 8·3 per cent of the marriages of schizophrenics. However, this particular sub-group was small and too much reliability cannot be attached to these crude estimates of complex emotional relations, especially in view of the large number of patients giving no causes for the breakdown of their marriages.

SUMMARY OF RESULTS ON SEPARATION AND DIVORCE

1. Before admission 17·9 per cent of ever married schizophrenics and 15·7 per cent of women suffering from affective disorders became separated or divorced from their first husbands; after admission 18·3 per cent of ever married schizophrenics experienced a separation or divorce which was a significantly higher proportion than the 10·2 per cent of women suffering from affective disorders who parted from their husbands (this was a significant difference at the one per cent level). At least 15 per cent of the patients in each clinical group had marriages of under 10 years' duration. In view of Rowntree's (1964) estimate that between 6·5 to 10·2 per cent of marriages of 10–20 years' duration end in separation or divorce in the general population, it would appear that schizophrenic women are especially liable to marital breakdown *before* and *after* their illness, and that women suffering from affective disorders are especially liable to such problems *before* their illness. The crucial factor in the marital breakdown of both clinical groups seemed to be the personality of the patients rather than factors specifically associated with their illness.

2. Analysis of frequency of separation and divorce by the relevant variables showed that during the period before admission patients in both clinical groups who married before the age of twenty were more likely to part from their husbands than those who married later and also in both clinical groups that patients with less than two children parted from their husbands more often than those having larger families; these findings tend to agree with those of Rowntree (1964) on women in the general population. The same clear differentials were not obtained for the period after admission.

3. Before admission, patients of both diagnoses who were described as normal personalities appeared a little less likely to part from their husbands than those exhibiting pronounced pre-morbid abnormalities, although the difference between these groups was not statistically significant.

4. After admission patients of both diagnoses who stayed in hospital longer

appeared to part from their husbands more frequently than those only staying for a short period, but these differences were only significant among schizophrenics.

5. Among those patients parting after admission, the illness itself did not appear to be the main cause of marital breakdown although little reliability can be attached to this particular aspect of the results.

6. Analysis of separation and divorce by religion and occupation produced results which were difficult to interpret. For example, there was some evidence suggesting that Roman Catholic patients parted from their husbands more frequently than Protestants in our sample of women suffering from affective disorders, but in view of lack of information on religion of husband and occupation no clear findings about the role of these variables in marital disruption could be stated.

CHAPTER XV

ILLEGITIMATE FERTILITY

INTRODUCTION

CASE records often contained detailed sexual histories from close relatives, friends, and the patient, and illegitimate births appeared to be given if they had occurred. For the purposes of this analysis the following two categories of illegitimate births were grouped together: (1) birth to single patients which were not legitimized by subsequent marriage to the child's father; and (2) births to 'ever married' patients, in cases where the father of the child was definitely given as a man other than the patient's husband.

Births to Jamaican patients which were the result of a stable cohabitation were considered illegitimate if there was no legal marriage. As in previous analyses [CHAPTERS X–XIV] it was decided to exclude the small group of patients suffering with serious physical illnesses associated with their mental state.

GENERAL RESULTS

TABLE 39 gives the number of illegitimate births per patient for the period before admission by their age at first illegitimate birth and clinical diagnosis.

TABLE 39

NUMBER OF PRE-PSYCHOTIC ILLEGITIMATE BIRTHS PER PATIENT BY DIAGNOSIS AND AGE AT FIRST BIRTH

Quinquennial age at 1st birth	Schizophrenics					Total no. of patients	Affectives					Total no. of patients
	Number of illegitimate births						Number of illegitimate births					
	1	2	3	4	5		1	2	3	4	5	
Under 15	1	–	–	–	–	1	–	–	–	–	–	–
15–19	11	6	–	–	1	18	6	4	–	–	–	10
20–24	22	4	1	1	2	30	13	–	–	–	–	13
25–29	8	–	–	–	–	8	2	1	–	–	–	3
30–34	6	–	–	–	–	6	1	1	–	1	–	3
35–39	4	–	–	–	–	4	3	1	–	–	–	4
40–44	1	–	–	–	–	1	1	–	–	–	–	1
N.K.	3	2	3	1	–	9	4	1	–	–	–	5
Total	56	12	4	2	3	77	30	8	–	1	–	39

Patients having no illegitimate births	720	439
Nothing known	16	4
Total sample	813	482

There were 115 such births to 813 schizophrenics; their mean age at first illegitimate birth was 23·7 (S.D. 6·2 years). The 482 women suffering from affective disorders had 50 illegitimate births, their mean age being 24·7 years (S.D. 7·2 years).

TABLE 40

NUMBER OF ILLEGITIMATE BIRTHS AFTER ADMISSION PER PATIENT BY AGE AT FIRST BIRTH AND DIAGNOSIS (EXCLUDING FOLLOW-UP DATA)

Age at first illeg. birth	Schizophrenics				Total no. of patients	Affectives				Total no. of patients
	No. of post-psychotic illeg. births					No. of post-psychotic illeg. births				
	1	2	3	4		1	2	3	4	
Under 15	1	–	–	–	1	–	–	–	–	–
15–19	4	–	–	–	4	–	–	–	–	–
20–24	8	–	1	–	9	2	–	–	–	2
25–29	5	–	–	–	5	–	–	–	–	–
30–34	4	1	–	–	5	–	–	–	–	–
35–39	1	–	–	–	1	–	1	–	–	1
40–44	2	–	–	–	2	–	–	–	–	–
Total	25	1	1	–	27	2	1	–	–	3

Total number having no illegitimate births	533	236
No data	11	2
No post-psychotic period	242	241
Total sample	813	482

There were fewer births during the period after admission up to last discharge [TABLE 40]: 571 schizophrenics observed during this period had 30 illegitimate children and their mean age at first illegitimate birth was 26·2 years (S.D. 7·5 years), whereas 241 women suffering from affective disorders only had four such births during this period. During the follow-up period 16 illegitimate births were found among the schizophrenics and four among the women suffering from affective disorders. Taking all periods of these patients' lives (both before and after admission) the 813 schizophrenics had 161 illegitimate children, and the 482 women suffering from affective disorders had 58 such children.

It is difficult to compare the two main clinical groups regarding illegitimate fertility; the schizophrenics were a younger group and owing to their low probability of marriage [CHAPTERS X and XI] more of them were exposed to the risk of an illegitimate conception. The women suffering from affective disorders were older and more had married, which accounted for the small numbers of illegitimate births after admission in this particular group. When births to single patients were analysed separately, during the period before first admission 43 of 370 schizophrenics, or 11·6 per cent, had at least one illegitimate child, and 13 out of 85 single women suffering from affective disorders (15·3 per cent). During the period after first admission (excluding follow-up data) 16 out of 252 schizophrenics (6·3 per cent) had at least one illegitimate child compared with only two of 35 single women with affective illnesses (5·7 per cent). These estimates are based on patients who were single on their last discharge from the hospital chosen, and do not include births to cohabiting patients who had previously been married.

Comparative data from the general population of England and Wales are generally based on synthetic cohorts which are difficult to relate to these results. In 1961 there were 17·2 illegitimate births per 1,000 single women of reproductive age, or 1·7 per 100 (General Register Office, 1963b). The percentage of single patients of reproductive age having an illegitimate child at any time up to the end of the follow-up appeared greatly in excess of the general population estimates but a real cohort of normal women is necessary to confirm this, and the group of single women with affective disorders was really too small to permit reliable statistical conclusions.

In order to overcome the problem of relating births in our cohort to estimates based on synthetic cohorts in the general population, it was decided to calculate the percentage of all live births in the sample which were illegitimate, compared with the percentage given for women in the general population. The schizophrenics had 682 legitimate and 161 illegitimate children, the percentage of total live births to schizophrenics which were illegitimate was therefore 19·1 per cent. The women who were suffering from affective disorders had 717 legitimate children and 58 illegitimate children, the percentage of their total live births which was illegitimate was 7·5 per cent. In 1961, 6 per cent of all live births were illegitimate in the general population of England and Wales. It would therefore appear that the schizophrenic women had a high illegitimate fertility whereas women suffering from affective disorders did not differ very significantly from women in the general population in this respect.

Since most of the illegitimate births to schizophrenics occurred before first admission, they could not be attributed solely to the effect of the illness in disturbing social and sexual inhibitions and diminishing responsibility. It seemed probable that the schizophrenics were more likely to have illegitimate births before admission than women in the general population because of their low probability of marriage during this period.

ANALYSIS OF ILLEGITIMATE FERTILITY BY SOCIO-PSYCHOLOGICAL VARIABLES

An attempt was made to relate illegitimate fertility in the sample to the relevant variables of interest in the opposite sex, race, personality, and social origins of the patients.

Interest in the Opposite Sex

Data were obtained for patients who were single on last discharge regarding their sexual relations, and interest in the opposite sex. During the period before admission most illegitimate births to schizophrenics appeared to be the result of an affair which was serious for the patient rather than the result of a casual sexual relationship. The women suffering from affective disorders had fewer illegitimate children, but a greater proportion of these appeared to be due to promiscuity than in the sample of schizophrenics. Most illegitimate births among the schizophrenics after admission did not appear to be due to casual relations with men, but there are too few births to women with affective illnesses to draw any tentative conclusions. These results demonstrate an interesting aspect of the lives of single schizophrenic women: although 28·6 of them had never been seriously involved with a man, *among* the 50·8 per cent of them that had at least one serious affair 22·3 per cent had an illegitimate child before admission, and 12·8 per cent after admission. Illegitimate fertility seemed high in this particular sub-group of single schizophrenic women.

Race

There were important racial differences in frequency of illegitimate births within each clinical group. Before their first admission 7·4 per cent of the 622 British white schizophrenics had at least one birth compared with 7·8 per cent of 399 women suffering from affective disorders who were British and white, 9·0 per cent of 122 non-British white schizophrenics had at least one child compared with 7·7 per cent of 65 women suffering from affective disorders in this group. Illegitimate births are most frequent among Jamaican patients, 43·6 per cent of 39 Jamaican schizophrenics, and 3 of the 7 Jamaican women with affective illnesses had illegitimate children. This is probably because stable cohabitation rather than legal marriage is a more frequent practice among this Jamaican group than among white patients.

During the period after admission the basic racial differentials in frequency of illegitimate births remained. There were too few births to women suffering from affective disorders to demonstrate this but 22·2 per cent of 27 Jamaican schizophrenics had an illegitimate child compared with only 3·1 per cent of 450 British white schizophrenics observed during this period. These estimates have assumed that the 'not knowns' had no illegitimate births and may therefore be taken as *conservative* estimates of illegitimate births to psychiatric patients.

Personality

During the period before admission the large group of 174 schizophrenics of schizoid personality had the lowest frequency of illegitimate children: only 6·3 per cent of them had at least one illegitimate child compared with 12·1 per cent of the group of 132 schizophrenic women whose personality was impossible to classify, this category included many possible psychopathic personalities. Among the women suffering from affective disorders 13·5 per cent of the 74 patients in the latter personality group had illegitimate children. Among patients having hitherto 'normal' personalities, 8·6 per cent of the 128

KMF

schizophrenics in this group and 3·5 per cent of the 115 women suffering from affective disorders in this category had at least one illegitimate child. These findings are perhaps very much as expected on psychological grounds, the schizoid patients are less likely to make serious heterosexual contacts, whereas normal personalities may do so but take precautions against illegitimate pregnancies, and patients with psychopathic tendencies may lack the responsibility to avoid such pregnancies. Generally, schizophrenics appeared more likely to have illegitimate children than women suffering from affective disorders whatever their personality type.

Most of the schizophrenics who had illegitimate children after admission appeared in the 'impossible to code some ?psychopathic category' of 83 patients, whereas all four such births to women with affective disorders were among those 54 patients in this clinical group having hitherto normal personalities. The numbers are really too small to allow meaningful analysis by type of personality.

Social Origin and Early Traumatic Events

The patients' fathers' occupations were taken as index of social origin. During the period before admission 9·2 per cent of the 413 schizophrenics giving information that their fathers were in manual occupations had an illegitimate child compared with only 4·8 per cent of those 169 with fathers in non-manual occupations. Among the women suffering from affective disorders 7 per cent of 257 patients with fathers in manual occupations and 11·4 per cent of 79 such women with fathers in non-manual work had at least one illegitimate child. After admission, 18 of 305 schizophrenic patients whose fathers were in manual occupations had at least one illegitimate child, whereas only one out of 111 patients with fathers in non-manual occupations had an illegitimate child. The 173 women suffering from affective disorders for whom there were data on the fathers' occupation, had no known illegitimate child. Little reliability can be attached to these particular results because for a very large number of cases in each clinical group there was no adequate information on the father's occupation (231 of 813 schizophrenics and 146 of 482 women with affective illnesses). Almost half of the illegitimate births before admission to schizophrenic women and women suffering from affective disorders were in this group, for which no adequate data were available about occupation of patient's father. It may well be that patients who are themselves illegitimate are more likely to have an illegitimate child, and that this is why half of such cases gave no details regarding their father's occupation.

An elementary attempt was made to assess the role of a disturbed childhood in producing behaviour leading to illegitimate births among our patients. A rough calculation was made for each main clinical group of the percentage *within* the group of patients having illegitimate children who had experienced the following trauma before the age of 21: discovery that they were illegitimate, separation of parents, death of one or both parents, or prolonged hospitalization of either parent. Considering all such traumatic events together, one-third of the schizophrenic women having illegitimate children had experienced such events, and just over a third of the women suffering from affective disorders had similar experiences.

It was decided that this particular aspect of the results required a special study requiring more time than was available during the period of the main study. In particular there was a need for intensive interviews not only with patients and their relatives, whether they had illegitimate births or not, but also a need for comparisons with samples drawn from the general population of England and Wales in order to reliably assess the significance of early psychic trauma in the development of behaviour leading to illegitimate children. The author hopes to undertake some further research in this particular area.

SUMMARY OF RESULTS ON ILLEGITIMATE FERTILITY

1. The 138 schizophrenic women had 161 illegitimate children, of whom only 46 were born after first admission. Their mean age at first birth before admission was $23 \cdot 7 \pm 6 \cdot 2$ years but for those having a birth after admission it was slightly higher ($26 \cdot 2 \pm 7 \cdot 5$ years).

2. The 482 women suffering from affective disorders had 58 illegitimate children, only eight of whom were born after admission; their mean age at first birth before admission was $24 \cdot 7 \pm 7 \cdot 3$ years, i.e. similar to that found for the schizophrenics. The low illegitimate fertility after admission among the women suffering from affective disorders was probably due to the fact that they were an older group on admission.

3. Of 370 single schizophrenics of reproductive age, $11 \cdot 6$ per cent had at least one illegitimate child before admission, and $6 \cdot 3$ per cent of 252 such women had an illegitimate child between first admission and last discharge. Of 85 single women suffering from affective disorders $15 \cdot 3$ per cent had at least one illegitimate child before admission. These percentages appear to be greatly in excess of the frequency of illegitimate births found in synthetic cohorts from the general population (there were $17 \cdot 2$ illegitimate births per 1,000 single women of reproductive age in 1961), but a real cohort of normal women in England and Wales is needed to make reliable comparisons with our patients.

4. Of the total live births to the schizophrenics $19 \cdot 1$ per cent were illegitimate, and $7 \cdot 5$ per cent of total births to women suffering from affective disorders were illegitimate, compared with 6 per cent of total live births being illegitimate in the general population in 1961. The illegitimate fertility of schizophrenics appeared to be high (perhaps because of their low probability of marriage), whereas that of women suffering from affective illnesses may not have been significantly different from the general population.

5. Half of the single schizophrenics had at least one affair which was serious

for the patient, and among this particular sub-group 22·3 per cent had an illegitimate child before admission and 12·8 per cent after. The data for women suffering from affective disorders by interest in the opposite sex were more difficult to interpret.

6. Illegitimate births were more frequent among Jamaican patients of both diagnoses than among white patients.

7. Among the schizophrenics, patients of schizoid personality had the lowest frequency of illegitimate births and patients whose personality was 'impossible to code and ?psychopathic' had the highest frequency. The latter group among the women suffering from affective disorders also had the highest frequency of illegitimate births.

8. It was impossible to analyse satisfactorily illegitimate births by social origin of the patient because about half of the patients having such births before admission gave no data on the occupation of the patient's father. This may be due to the fact that about one-third of the patients in each main clinical group who had illegitimate children either were themselves illegitimate or had experienced severely traumatic events during their childhood, such as separation of parents or death or prolonged hospitalization of either parent.

A brief comparison of the above findings in relation to the relevant literature on unmarried mothers is given in CHAPTER XVIII; most studies appear to have been undertaken in the United States.

CHAPTER XVI

MISCELLANEOUS DATA

IN the course of this survey some additional information was obtained on the following topics: (1) assortative mating; (2) infertility; (3) cause of death; (4) parental age; (5) mental illness in the family.

As in previous analyses, it was decided to exclude patients who were suffering from a severe physical illness associated with their mental state.

ASSORTATIVE MATING

Eleven of 440 ever married schizophrenic women, or 2·5 per cent, had husbands who were also mentally ill, compared with 4·9 per cent of the 386 ever married women suffering from affective disorders. TABLE 41 gives the

TABLE 41

MENTAL ILLNESS IN THE HUSBANDS OF PATIENTS BY DIAGNOSIS OF HUSBAND AND PATIENT

Husband's diagnosis	Diagnosis of female patients in sample	
	Schizophrenic n = 440 ever married patients	Affective disorder n = 386 ever married patients
Schizophrenia	1	2
Manic-depressive	2	4
Neurotic reactions	–	4
Suicide or attempted suicide	2	4
Drug addiction	–	1
Alcoholism	–	1
Mental deficiency	1	–
Organic brain disease	3	2
Not known	2	1
Total	11	19

diagnosis of the 30 husbands for whom there was this information for each main clinical group of patients. There appeared to be a higher incidence of functional disorders among the husbands of women suffering from affective disorders than among the husbands of schizophrenics. These figures were based solely on cases in which there was very definite evidence of mental disorder in the husband, such as an admission or out-patient treatment, and therefore they did not include unstable and peculiar personalities among husbands. The case records were read in order to discover whether the husband's illness appeared to be a reaction to that of our patient: only two

husbands of the schizophrenics and three husbands of the women suffering from affective disorders appeared to have become ill in this way; on the
other hand, the data suggested that there were more cases where the patient
had become ill or deteriorated as a result of the husband's illness. However, in
view of the complexity of marital relationships too much reliability could not
be attached to this finding.

The amount of assortative mating is somewhat lower than would be
expected among the schizophrenics when compared with MacSorley's (1964)
result that 5·1 per cent of female patients were married to mentally-ill husbands. Our women suffering from affective disorders, however, appeared very
similar to MacSorley's sample in this respect, i.e. 4·9 per cent. Controlled
comparisons were difficult because MacSorley's sample contained some
patients suffering from organic psychoses. Possibly our sample represents a
low estimate of assortative mating for some reason associated with the fact
that it is a sample of women. MacSorley found a considerably higher incidence
of mental illness among the wives of male patients (13 per cent).

INFERTILITY

The schizophrenics appeared to have a slightly higher proportion of infertile marriages than the women suffering from affective disorders [TABLE 42];
this may be partly because the schizophrenics were younger and their families
were less complete, or because there are more cases where definite evidence of
fertility was not given (as in the paranoid group). According to the 1951
Census Fertility Report (General Register Office 1959) 20 per cent of the
married women aged 45–9 and over were infertile and 80 per cent fertile
(Section C on completed fertility, Table C1, p. 178). Of the main group of
undifferentiated schizophrenics, 76·5 per cent were fertile, and 78·9 per cent
of the women suffering from affective disorders. In view of the fact that these
patients were of childbearing age, many of whose families were incomplete,
they did not appear to differ significantly from the general population in
infertility and the catatonic and schizo-affective patients appeared to demonstrate low infertility.

There was inadequate information on cause of infertility but definite
physical reasons were given for more patients with paranoid schizophrenia
than for other clinical groups.

CAUSE OF DEATH

TABLE 43 shows that suicide accounted for over half the known deaths in
our sample of women of childbearing age. Sixteen (2 per cent) of the 813
schizophrenics had committed suicide, their mean age at death was 33·9 years;
19 of the 482 women suffering from affective disorders (3·9 per cent) had
committed suicide, their mean age at death was higher at 41·1 years, probably
because of the later onset of affective disorders.

These findings tended to agree with those of previous studies in other

TABLE 42

FOR EVER MARRIED PATIENTS ON LAST DISCHARGE: REASONS FOR INFERTILITY BY DIAGNOSIS

Diagnosis	N/A i.e. fertile marriages %	Physical reasons			Sexual difficulties %	Involuntary cause N.K. %	Not married long enough %	Choice %	N.K. %	Total N
		Ovarian factors %	Seminal factors %	Other %						
Schizophrenia	76·5	1·5	1·1	1·5	3·0	3·0	3·0	2·2	8·2	268
Paranoid	64·6	5·3	1·8	2·7	1·8	3·5	–	4·4	15·9	113
Catatonic	85·0	–	–	–	–	–	5·0	–	10·0	20
Schizo-affective	81·0	2·4	–	2·4	4·8	2·4	–	2·4	4·8	42
Affective	78·9	1·5	0·8	–	1·5	4·9	0·5	4·1	7·7	388
Total	76·4	2·0	1·0	1·0	2·2	3·9	1·3	3·4	8·9	831

TABLE 43

CAUSE OF DEATH BY DIAGNOSIS

Diagnosis	Neoplasms	Vascular lesions affecting nervous system	Heart disease	Cause of death Pneumonia and influenza	Other	Suicide	Homicide	N.K.
Schizophrenia	2	–	1	4	–	12	1	6
Paranoid	1	–	–	1	–	2	–	–
Catatonic	–	1	–	1	–	–	–	–
Schizo-affective	–	–	–	1	–	3	–	–
Affective	1	–	–	2	1	18	1	5
Total	4	1	1	9	1	35	2	11

countries: the percentage of schizophrenics who commit suicide always appears to be far below that found for manic-depressives. First, in respect of the schizophrenics, Rupp and Fletcher (1939–40) followed up 641 patients for 5–10 years and found that 1·96 per cent had committed suicide compared with 5·9 per cent found by Fremming (1951) in a Danish survey, and 2·3 per cent given by Helgason (1964) in his Icelandic survey. Both of the later estimates followed up the patients until they were over the age of 50. The corresponding percentage of manic-depressives who committed suicide was 11 per cent (Fremming, 1951) and 17·4 per cent (Helgason, 1964). Presumably our estimates were lower than these because of some lack of information about cause of death during the follow-up, and because our sample was of women of childbearing age, who are less likely to commit suicide than men or older age groups of either sex (Sainsbury, 1955).

The risk of suicide in both clinical groups (2–4 per cent) would appear to be considerably greater than that found in the general population. In Kensington, which is part of the catchment area, Sainsbury found a high suicide rate compared with other London areas, i.e. 7·4 per 100,000 women aged 15–34, and 26·6 per 100,000 women aged 35–54 in 1931 or much less than 0·5 per cent. Recent estimates for conurbations give the rate for women aged 15 and over as 128 per million or 0·013 per cent (General Register Office 1964).

PARENTAL AGE

The mean age at patient's birth of her mother was 30·1 years for the schizophrenics (S.D. 6·58 years), and 30·22 years for the women suffering from affective disorders (S.D. 6·8 years) [TABLE 44]. The mean age of the patient's

TABLE 44

MOTHER'S AGE AT BIRTH OF PATIENT BY DIAGNOSIS

Diagnosis	Mother's age in quinquennial groups							N.K.	N
	Under 20	20–4	25–9	30–4	35–9	40–4	45–9		
Schizophrenia	14	61	93	77	49	24	2	213	533
Paranoid	5	16	29	17	15	5	1	84	172
Catatonic	1	1	10	6	3	3	–	15	39
Schizo-affective	2	5	13	10	7	2	–	30	69
Affective disorder	12	51	73	70	42	20	2	212	482
Total	34	134	218	180	116	54	5	554	1295

father at this time was a little higher, i.e. 34·6 years (S.D. 7·83) for the schizophrenics and 33·27 years (S.D. 7·84 years) for the women suffering from affective disorders [TABLE 45]. 13·7 per cent of the mothers of the schizophrenics (excluding schizo-affectives) and 13·2 per cent of the mothers of the women with affective disorders were known to be aged 35 or over at the birth of the patient, which was a lower proportion than would be expected on the basis of the general population, i.e. since 1900 the proportion of all mothers

TABLE 45

FATHER'S AGE AT BIRTH OF PATIENT BY DIAGNOSIS

Diagnosis	Father's age in quinquennial groups									N.K.	N
	15–19	20–4	25–9	30–4	35–9	40–4	45–9	50–4	55+		
Schizophrenia	2	19	49	74	52	29	22	8	2	276	533
Paranoid	1	4	22	16	10	6	5	–	1	107	172
Catatonic	1	–	3	7	3	2	–	–	1	22	39
Schizo-affective	–	5	4	9	7	2	4	–	–	38	69
All affective states	5	23	63	55	43	31	9	2	4	247	482
Total	9	51	141	161	115	70	40	10	8	690	1295

in these older age groups has varied from 22 per cent for 1901–5 to 17 per cent for 1936–40 (Goodman, 1957). Even if the calculation of the proportion of older mothers was limited to case notes giving this information, the proportion only reached 23·7 per cent. The results therefore tended to agree with those of Granville-Grossman (1966) in finding no definite evidence for advanced maternal age at the birth of schizophrenic patients, and did not agree with Goodman's data suggesting support from this increased maternal age (1957).

MENTAL ILLNESS IN THE FAMILY:*
PARENTS OF OUR PATIENTS

The Schizophrenic Sample

At least 15·3 per cent of either of the parents of the 744 schizophrenic women had suffered from some form of functional mental disorder. This proportion included cases in which the parent may not have been admitted to mental hospitals. Unfortunately, the information on mental illness among relatives was not considered to be very reliable: 15 per cent of the records of each main clinical group gave no details about mental illness among parents, 70 per cent of the records of the schizophrenics definitely denied any mental illness among the parents.

Considering incidence of specific psychoses among parents, only 1·75 per cent of the schizophrenic women had parents who were definitely known to have also suffered from schizophrenia; there appeared to be more mothers with this disorder, namely ten compared with only three fathers. It would appear likely that this was a serious underestimation of the true frequency of schizophrenia among the parents of women in this clinical group, because of lack of detailed family histories. Previous studies have suggested that between 5 and 12 per cent of the parents of schizophrenics have also suffered from schizophrenia (Luxenburger, 1935; Kallmann, 1946; Böök, 1953; Zerbin-Rüdin, 1963). Shields and Slater (1967) give a pooled estimate of 5·07 per cent. A special study was really required in order to assess incidence of schizophrenia among the parents of patients whose records gave no evidence of this, but this was unfortunately not possible during the period allowed for this survey.

With regard to incidence of affective disorders among the parents of schizophrenic women, 2·3 per cent of the patients had one parent who had suffered from these illnesses: in two cases both parents had experienced an affective disorder; in 14 cases mothers fall into this group and in nine cases the fathers. Again, there would appear to be a preponderance of mothers rather than fathers with functional mental disorders. In view of the low reliability of this aspect of the data, no attempt was made to calculate morbid risks among the parents of schizophrenics by any sophisticated techniques.

* The 69 women suffering from schizo-affective disorders were excluded from these calculations, in view of their probably mixed genetic aetiology.

Women Suffering from Affective Illnesses

At least 11·9 per cent of the 482 women in this clinical group had parents who had suffered from some form of functional mental disorder. However, as mentioned above, in 15 per cent of the records of this group there was also no information on parents' mental illness, and 71·8 per cent of this group gave definite evidence against such illness among parents. There was not one case of schizophrenia found among the parents of patients suffering from affective disorders. Four mothers and three fathers of such patients, or 1·4 per cent of the 482 women in this group, were known to have parents who suffered from an affective illness. As in the schizophrenic group, it appeared likely that this was a serious underestimation of true incidence among parents, and in view of lack of information about diagnosis of parents, and complete lack of data in so many cases it was decided not to analyse any further this particular aspect of the research.

MENTAL ILLNESS AMONG THE SIBS OF THE PATIENTS

Schizophrenic Sample

Of the schizophrenic women 7·1 per cent had at least one sib who had suffered from some form of functional mental disorder. Unfortunately, such information was missing in about a quarter of the patients' records, and the records of 488 out of 744 patients, or well over 60 per cent, contained a denial of mental illness in the sibships. In respect of schizophrenia itself, only 2·6 per cent of the sibs of the schizophrenics were known to have actually had a schizophrenic illness. This was a surprisingly low proportion in view of previous estimates that frequency of schizophrenia among the sibs of schizophrenic patients is between 5 and 14 per cent (Slater and Shields, 1953; Garrone, 1962). More recently Shields and Slater (1967) gave a pooled estimate of 8·53 per cent. It should be remembered that many of the apparently normal sibs of our women of reproductive age may eventually develop schizophrenia, but in view of the lack of reliable information it was decided to refrain from any further analysis of this problem. Of the schizophrenics 1·3 per cent were found to have sibs who had an affective illness.

As in the estimates of illness among parents, women with schizo-affective disorders were excluded from these estimates.

The Sample of Women Suffering from Affective Disorders

Of these women 6·9 per cent were found to have sibs who had some form of functional mental illness. In spite of the lack of information in 26·1 per cent of the 482 patients' records and the fact that 53·9 per cent denied any such illness in the sibs, 3·4 per cent of the patients had sibs who definitely also experienced an affective illness. Only 0·6 per cent of the affectives had sibs who were known to develop a schizophrenic illness. It therefore appears that incidence of the same type of illness as the patients' is higher among the sibs in each main group than alternative forms of mental disorders, indicating possibly some differential genetic basis for each clinical group.

Little reliability can be attached to these results on mental illness among parents and sibs of our patients because of the lack of information given in case histories.

SUMMARY OF ADDITIONAL FINDINGS

1. Of the ever married schizophrenics 2·5 per cent, and of the women suffering from affective disorders 4·9 per cent, had husbands who were also mentally ill. The main forms of disorder among these husbands were depressive reactions, including suicides, but this did not generally appear to be a result of stress associated with the patient's illness. The amount of assortative mating appeared low among the schizophrenics but similar to that expected among the women with affective disorders when compared with MacSorley's (1964) data on a group of patients suffering from both functional and organic disorders.

2. The number of infertile marriages in both clinical groups did not appear to differ significantly from that expected on the basis of the general population.

3. Suicide accounts for over half the deaths in the sample: 2 per cent of the schizophrenics committed suicide, and 3·9 per cent of the women suffering from affective disorders. There were probably some undiscovered suicides, as these proportions are lower than would be expected on the basis of previous studies, especially for the latter clinical group. The risk of suicide in both clinical groups was far greater than that found in the general population.

4. No evidence could be found for advanced maternal age at birth of the schizophrenics nor for the women suffering from affective disorders.

5. There was a lack of reliable information in case records on mental illness among the parents and sibs of the patients. Crude proportions of patients in each main clinical group showed definite evidence of such illness among their relatives, indicating a tendency to increased risks of mental illness within the family; the quality of information was too poor to enable any reliable statistical estimates.

CHAPTER XVII

RELIABILITY OF DATA

RELIABILITY OF PSYCHIATRIC DIAGNOSIS

FOR the purposes of the analysis it was decided to accept the last diagnosis made by a consultant at the hospital chosen for sampling. In order to assess the reliability of this diagnosis Dr. J. K. Wing, Director of the Medical Research Council Social Psychiatry Research Unit, examined a sub-sample of case notes. A 5 per cent random sample of the final total sample of 1,325 was selected by picking out every twentieth patient; Dr. Wing read the clinical notes of the 63 patients thus selected and made his own diagnosis. TABLE 46 relates the original diagnosis to his.

In 65 per cent of the patients Dr. Wing agreed with the diagnosis accepted and a further 14 cases involved changes within our main *clinical* groups which would not affect the validity of the special analysis of marriage and fertility, so that 87·3 per cent of this sub-sample were considered to be reliable diagnoses. In only 16 per cent was there a diagnostic change away from the main categories: within this group, there were only two changes to a totally unrelated diagnostic group, i.e. one epileptic psychosis and the other personality disorder. Other changes involved queries regarding type of puerperal psychosis.

Dr. Wing considered that the acceptance of the consultant's diagnosis was adequate for the purposes of this study and that the main clinical groups, namely the schizophrenics and the women suffering from affective disorders, were reliable classifications.

TABLE 46

RELATIONSHIP BETWEEN DIAGNOSIS ACCEPTED AND INDEPENDENT
DIAGNOSIS MADE FROM CLINICAL NOTES

Changes from original diagnosis	*Number of patients*
No change	41
Change within the schizophrenias	11
Change within the affective states	3
Change from schizophrenia to affectives	3
Change from affectives to schizophrenia	1
Other changes, including not knowns	4
Total	63

Inter-hospital Study of Diagnostic Change

A further check on the reliability of the accepted diagnosis was made by writing to all other hospitals in which each patient had been treated in order to discover whether there had been previous and independent diagnoses different from that accepted in this survey. Such clinical information was found for 305 single schizophrenic women, for 349 ever married patients of this diagnosis, for 77 single women suffering from affective disorders and for 262 ever married patients in the latter clinical group. The marital status referred to here was that given on the admission from which they were selected into the sample.

Over 70 per cent of each main clinical and marital status category involved no change in diagnosis. Only 10·5 per cent of the single schizophrenics and 13·5 per cent of the married ones had ever had a diagnosis within the category of affective disorders. A further 9·6 per cent of the single schizophrenics, and 5·7 per cent of the married ones had a change of diagnosis to another clinical category such as personality disorder.

The women suffering from affective disorders showed a slightly higher percentage of change to other diagnoses; 10·4 per cent of these women who were single, and 8·4 per cent of those who were married, had been diagnosed as schizophrenic at some time. A further 18·2 per cent of the 77 single women with affective disorders, and 14·5 per cent of the 262 married ones had also been diagnosed as suffering from other forms of mental disorder such as anxiety neurosis or psychopathic personality, which were not the main diagnoses allowed in the main sample. It should be emphasized that this does not necessarily mean that the diagnosis accepted in our survey was unreliable; for example, the women suffering from affective disorders may have hitherto been suffering from a severe anxiety state or personality disorder, and still have a severe depression when admitted to the hospital chosen for sampling or they may have experienced a subsequent breakdown in which an alternative diagnosis was possible. It was concluded that for the purposes of this survey the diagnoses accepted are at least 70 per cent reliable.

ACCURACY OF INFORMATION

TABLE 47 shows how at least two thirds of the case histories came from a source other than the patient herself. There was, however, an important difference by diagnosis: in only 6–8 per cent of the schizophrenic groups was the patient herself the only source of information, whereas 29·3 per cent of the women with affective disorders fell into this category. *This difference was statistically significant at the 1 per cent level.* This was probably because the women with affective disorders contained a large proportion of women who were not deluded, and who could give their own histories, whereas the schizophrenics were often too disturbed for this.

Considering other sources of information: the husbands and parents of

TABLE 47

SOURCE OF INFORMATION BY DIAGNOSIS

Source of information (percentage distribution)

Diagnosis	Husband	Husband + parent(s)	Parents only: married pts	Parents only: single pts	Relatives + G.P.	Relatives + Other hospitals	Relatives + welfare agencies	Welfare agencies only	Hospital + welfare	Patient only	N.K.	Total N
Schizophrenia	10·7	6·8	5·1	16·5	23·8	8·1	8·8	3·9	6·6	6·8	3·0	533
Paranoid	15·7	2·9	5·2	8·1	22·1	9·3	9·9	5·2	8·1	9·3	4·1	172
Catatonic	5·1	2·6	5·1	17·9	33·3	7·7	7·7	5·1	5·1	7·7	2·6	39
Schizo-affective	15·9	8·7	5·8	15·9	17·4	11·6	5·8	1·4	7·2	8·7	1·4	69
Affectives	20·1	3·7	5·4	4·6	11·8	11·4	4·4	2·7	2·5	29·3	4·1	482
Total	15·0	5·1	5·3	11·0	19·1	9·7	7·1	3·6	5·3	15·6	3·5	1295

married women suffering from affective illnesses gave slightly more data than the corresponding relatives of married schizophrenics. However, general practitioners and welfare agencies gave more data on schizophrenics than on the women with affective disorders, probably because the schizophrenics had more contact with their doctors or welfare workers. We may conclude from TABLE 47 that the data obtained for the analysis should be reliable.

NON-RESPONSE BIAS

In order to assess whether the results on marriage and fertility after admission were biassed by the 20 per cent non-response to the follow-up inquiry, it was decided to tabulate whether the patients were traced or not during the follow-up by the following relevant variables: (1) personality; (2) length of stay in hospital; (3) marital status; (4) social class by husband's occupation; (5) religion; and (6) race.

Personality

In CHAPTER XI it was demonstrated that the probability of marriage of schizophrenic women after admission was significantly reduced, especially among those patients of schizoid personality. If this type of patient was especially difficult to trace during the follow-up, it could have meant the follow-up sample was biassed towards those schizophrenics who were more likely to marry than the schizoid patients. TABLE 48 shows how the non-response rate for schizoid patients was always well below 20 per cent, i.e. below the average rate for the entire sample, and therefore our results on probability of marriage after admission would not overestimate this by some bias towards more extraverted schizophrenics. Patients of normal personality did not appear to be easy to trace. A very small group of 22 single women with affective disorders, who were considered to be of a normal pre-morbid temperament, had a 36 per cent non-response rate. Single women with affective disorders were generally the most difficult group to trace. However, the role of personality appeared less important among the women suffering from affective illnesses and these women did not differ significantly from the general population in probability of marriage.

More schizophrenics stayed in hospital compared with women with affective disorders; 17·6 per cent of the single schizophrenics and 12·5 per cent of the married ones were known to be in hospital or to have died in hospital by the time of the follow-up inquiry, compared with only 4·3 per cent of the single women with affective disorders, and 4·9 per cent of the married women in this clinical group. Of those schizophrenics who were discharged there was slightly more response from general practitioners, hospitals, and welfare agencies, whereas among the women with affective disorders the patients or their families seemed to reply more to the postal follow-up. This finding, of course, mirrors the basic finding from information in case records, i.e. that women with affective disorders tended to give more

LMF

TABLE 48

METHOD OF TRACING PATIENTS DURING THE FOLLOW-UP BY PERSONALITY, DIAGNOSIS AND MARITAL STATUS

Method of tracing patient (percentage distribution)

Personality	Schizophrenics — Single By pt or rel. %	By G.P. hosp. welfare %	Still in hosp. or died in hosp. %	N.T.* %	N	Schizophrenics — Married By pt or rel. %	By G.P. hosp. welfare %	Still in hosp. or died in hosp. %	N.T. %	N	Affectives — Single By pt or rel. %	By G.P. hosp. welfare %	Still in hosp. or died in hosp. %	N.T. %	N	Affectives — Married By pt or rel. %	By G.P. hosp. welfare %	Still in hosp. or died in hosp. %	N.T. %	N
Schizoid	16·5	46·9	22·0	14·7	109	27·7	44·6	10·8	16·9	65	53·9	38·5	-	7·7	13	40·0	31·1	8·9	20·0	45
Prone to variable moods	5·8	49·9	23·5	20·6	34	23·1	36·5	21·2	19·2	52	-	54·6	18·2	27·3	11	28·6	45·3	7·1	19·0	42
Neurotic	-	49·9	14·3	35·7	14	42·2	46·6	4·4	6·7	45	25·1	43·9	-	31·3	16	33·6	41·3	4·8	20·6	63
Combination	23·1	53·7	12·8	10·3	39	23·8	45·2	11·9	19·0	42	100·0	-	-	-	3	17·7	58·8	8·8	14·7	34
Impossible to code—includes psychopathic	20·3	44·4	13·9	21·5	79	34·6	26·9	15·4	23·1	52	15·0	50·0	5·0	30·0	20	26·0	48·2	3·7	22·2	54
Normal	20·0	40·1	20·0	20·0	35	32·3	46·4	8·6	12·9	93	13·6	45·3	4·5	36·4	22	44·1	35·5	3·2	17·2	93
Not known	11·3	46·7	13·3	26·7	60	13·2	47·3	15·4	24·2	91	11·1	44·6	-	44·4	9	27·3	47·2	1·8	23·6	55
Total	16·2	46·9	17·6	19·5	370	27·0	42·7	12·5	17·7	440	22·3	44·7	4·3	28·7	94	32·9	42·4	4·9	19·7	386

* N.T. = Not traced in this and subsequent tabulations.

information themselves, than schizophrenics, probably because more of the former group have insight into their disorder.

Length of Hospital Stay

Long stays in hospital appeared to be important in reducing probability of marriage after admission of schizophrenics [CHAPTER XI] and in reducing legitimate fertility after admission in both clinical groups [CHAPTER XIII]. TABLE 49 shows how short-stay cases involved more non-response than long-stay patients in both single and married schizophrenics and among the married women with affective disorders. This was partly due to the fact that more long-stay cases were in the same hospital at the time of follow-up and therefore were very easy to trace. This could mean a slight underestimation of marriage and fertility after admission, because the follow-up sample was slightly biassed towards more chronic cases. This has been dealt with in the special fertility analysis which controlled for hospitalization, and demonstrated that most reductions in fertility after admission were largely dependent on hospitalization.

Marital Status

TABLE 50 shows how among the schizophrenics the single and married patients were easier to trace than those who were separated or widowed. Among the women with affective disorders the small group of single women were especially difficult to trace, probably because they are a mobile group who do not make so much contact with hospitals and welfare agencies; the married women with affective disorders were easier to trace than the separated or divorced, but unlike the schizophrenics the widowed in this group had a low non-response rate. These findings indicate that (1) we may have underestimated probability of marriage of women with affective disorders, although this did not appear to differ significantly from the general population; and (2) that the analysis of marital status changes had omitted some remarriages because divorced and separated patients were difficult to trace.

It would appear that these biases did not seriously affect the results of the special analysis of marriage and fertility, especially in view of the fact that the two groups who exhibited important differentials, namely, the single and married schizophrenics, had comparatively low non-response rates, 19·5 and 15·4 per cent respectively.

Social Class by Husband's Occupation

Of the schizophrenics married to manual workers, 15·6 per cent could not be traced compared with 12·1 per cent in the non-manual group. This was partly compensated by the fact that 17·7 per cent of the schizophrenics married to manual workers were in hospital at the time of the follow-up, compared with only 6·5 per cent of those women who were married to non-manual workers. There did not seem to be such differences by social class of

TABLE 49

METHOD OF TRACING PATIENT DURING THE FOLLOW-UP BY TOTAL LENGTH OF HOSPITAL STAY ON DISCHARGE

| | Schizophrenics | | | | | | | | | | Affectives | | | | | | | | | |
| | Single | | | | | Married | | | | | Single | | | | | Married | | | | |
Length of stay	By pt or rel. %	By G.P. hosp. welfare %	Still in hosp. or died in hosp. %	N.T. %	N	By pt or rel. %	By G.P. hosp. welfare %	Still in hosp. or died in hosp. %	N.T. %	N	By pt or rel. %	By G.P. hosp. welfare %	Still in hosp. or died in hosp. %	N.T. %	N	By pt or rel. %	By G.P. hosp. welfare %	Still in hosp. or died in hosp. %	N.T. %	N
Up to 12 months	17·5	52·6	4·6	25·3	194	28·7	45·9	5·3	20·1	284	25·0	48·5	–	26·5	68	34·8	41·8	3·2	20·9	316
1–10+ years	13·6	37·9	40·9	7·6	132	24·6	35·4	27·7	12·3	130	18·0	27·0	27·0	27·0	11	20·0	52·5	25·0	2·5	40
Not known	22·9	47·7	0·5	29·5	44	19·0	47·0	16·0	19·0	26	13·3	40·0	6·7	40·0	15	29·9	36·7	3·3	30·0	30
Total	16·2	46·9	17·6	19·5	370	27·0	42·7	12·5	17·7	440	22·3	44·7	4·3	28·7	94	32·9	42·4	4·9	19·7	386

TABLE 50

METHOD OF TRACING PATIENT DURING THE FOLLOW-UP BY MARITAL STATUS ON LAST DISCHARGE

Marital status	Schizophrenics					Affectives				
	Pt or rel. %	G.P., hosp. or welfare %	In hosp. or died %	N.T. %	N	Pt or rel. %	G.P., hosp. or welfare %	In hosp. or died %	N.T. %	N
Single	16·1	47·7	18·1	19·2	360	23·9	42·8	3·6	29·8	84
Cohabiting	20·0	50·0	–	30·0	10	10·0	60·0	10·0	20·0	10
Married	28·4	43·3	13·0	15·4	324	34·2	43·1	4·2	18·5	313
Married but separated	16·0	42·8	12·5	28·8	56	24·2	42·7	6·1	27·3	33
Divorced	32·5	40·0	10·0	17·5	40	26·0	34·6	8·7	30·4	23
Widowed	25·0	40·0	10·0	25·0	20	35·3	41·3	11·8	11·8	17
Total	22·1	44·6	14·8	18·5	810	30·8	42·9	4·8	21·4	480

husband among the women with affective disorders. We could not trace 18·7 per cent of the women in this group who were married to manual workers, nor 19·2 per cent of those married to non-manual workers. The highest non-response rates are among those patients in each clinical group whose husband's occupation was not known, 29·2 per cent of the schizophrenics and 21·9 per cent of the women with affective disorders in the latter category could not be traced. This category contained a high proportion of women who have parted from their husbands [see CHAPTER XIV].

The follow-up inquiry did not appear to produce any social class bias which could seriously affect the analysis of legitimate fertility after admission.

Religion

Roman Catholics were more difficult to trace in both clinical groups than Church of England and Nonconformist groups. Of the 99 schizophrenic women who were Roman Catholics, 25·3 per cent could not be traced compared with 17·9 per cent of the 28 patients in this clinical group who were Nonconformists, and only 15·8 per cent of the 292 schizophrenics belonging to the Church of England. Among the women with affective illnesses, 26·3 per cent of the 95 Roman Catholics could not be traced, compared with 16·7 per cent of 24 Nonconformists and 17·4 per cent of 253 women belonging to the Church of England within this group. This was probably due to the fact that a large proportion of the Roman Catholics were Irish or Polish immigrants who are perhaps more mobile or who do not completely understand letters sent to them. Since a special analysis was undertaken of the marriage and fertility of British white patients this source of bias should not seriously influence the results.

Race

The British whites had the lowest non-response rate in all clinical groups. The relationship between non-response and race was most clearly demonstrated in the single schizophrenics. Among this particular group 55·6 per cent of the 27 schizophrenic Negresses could not be traced, compared with 29·5 per cent of the 61 non-British whites, and only 12·9 per cent of the 272 British whites. Among the married schizophrenics, a quarter of 20 Negresses could not be traced, 32·8 per cent of 61 non-British whites, but only 15 per cent of 347 British white patients were not traced.

Of the single women with affective disorders, 3 out of 5 Negresses and 58·8 per cent of 17 non-British whites were not traced, but only 19·7 per cent of 71 British whites could not be found. Lastly, within the category of 386 married women with affective disorders, there were only 4 Negresses, one of whom could not be traced, but 23·4 per cent of 47 non-British white patients were not found, compared with the lower non-response rate of 19 per cent for the 327 British white women in this group. *These figures emphasized the importance of race as a variable in sociological analysis and gave added reason for the separate analysis undertaken of British white patients* [see CHAPTERS X and XI on marriage, and CHAPTERS XII and XIII on fertility].

SUMMARY OF ASSESSMENT OF RELIABILITY OF DATA

1. The main diagnosis accepted in the survey was considered to be at least 80 per cent reliable by an independent consultant after his inspection of a 5 per cent random sub-sample of patients' clinical notes. A separate inter-hospital check on previous or subsequent diagnoses for as many patients as possible also indicated that the diagnosis accepted was 70 per cent reliable.

2. Over 90 per cent of the case histories of the schizophrenics contained detailed information from a source other than the patient, whereas only 70 per cent of the notes of women suffering from affective illnesses had such an independent source of information. This may have been due to the fact that a considerable proportion of women with affective disorders were suffering from reactive depressions, and since they were not deluded they were more reliable informants than the schizophrenics. Data from both clinical groups were considered reliable for the purposes of analysing probability of marriage and legitimate fertility.

3. (a) The 20 per cent non-response to the postal follow-up inquiry did not result in any bias of personality types which could seriously affect the results on probability of marriage after admission.

   (b) Short-stay cases appeared more difficult to follow up than long-stay patients, and this could lead to a slight underestimation of probability of marriage after admission. The role of hospitalization on fertility after admission was carefully assessed so that no such bias in the follow-up could seriously influence the results.

   (c) Among the schizophrenics, married women were easier to trace than separated patients, or single patients in this clinical group. Single women suffering from affective disorders were especially difficult to trace, as were divorced and separated patients in this clinical group. This could mean some slight underestimation of marriage, after admission, especially among the women with affective illnesses.

   (d) Higher non-response among the schizophrenics, who were wives of manual workers, was compensated by the fact that more patients in this particular sub-category were in hospital at the time of follow-up and there did not appear to be any serious bias in terms of social class which could affect the results on fertility.

   (e) Roman Catholics were more difficult to trace than other Christian patients, and this was linked with the fact that non-British white patients, who were mainly Roman Catholic, were difficult to trace compared with British white patients. Coloured patients were also more difficult to trace. This source of bias could have lead to some underestimation of fertility after admission but the separate analysis of British white patients excluded the effect of racial variations on fertility.

In conclusion, the 20 per cent non-response did not appear to involve any serious bias in the main results. There was the possibility of some slight underestimation of probability of marriage after admission, especially among the women suffering from affective disorders. However, it appears unlikely that this particular group of women would demonstrate any really significant differentials when compared with women in the corresponding general population.

Part 5. Discussion and Conclusions

CHAPTER XVIII

DISCUSSION OF RESULTS IN RELATION TO THOSE OF PREVIOUS STUDIES

INTRODUCTION

SINCE the earlier investigations there have been such profound clinical and social changes that it is difficult to compare results obtained from patients living in different countries at different times. In particular, the advent of tranquillizing and other psychiatric drugs since 1954 has produced a revolution in the treatment of severely disturbed patients: the typical picture of long-term institutional care has been replaced by community psychiatry involving both the patient and her family. From the sociological viewpoint the spread of birth control to all social classes, and post-war economic development have lessened differential fertility within Western countries. These major clinical and social trends have reduced the social differences between the lives of psychiatric patients and normal women and this is mirrored in the diminishing of marriage and fertility differentials.

PROBABILITY OF MARRIAGE BEFORE ADMISSION

First, considering the results on probability of marriage before admission [CHAPTER XI], the reduction within the schizophrenic group to 73·4±2·6 per cent of normal would appear to be in the expected direction when compared with cruder estimates of proportions ever married on first admission such as those of Popenoe (1928a) in California, Nissen (1932) in Scandinavia, Kallmann (1938) in Berlin, and Böök (1953) in a north Swedish isolate. Comparisons with Essen-Möller's (1935) Bavarian sample were especially difficult. Our findings agree with his in direction in that there was a marked reduction in the probability of marriage of schizophrenic women before admission, but no exact estimate could be derived from his data, since he has subsequently suggested (Essen-Möller, 1967, personal communication) that his correction for the under-representation of the married in hospital was overdone. More recently, Ødegaard (1960) gave evidence that the marriage rate of schizophrenic women admitted to Norwegian hospitals between 1946 and 1955 was only 56·6 per cent of that expected in the corresponding general population, which appears considerably lower than our estimate, which controlled for age at and date of admission, and was based on a more recent admission sample, namely 1955–63. The differentials between patients and women in the general population seem to have lessened considerably. Erlenmeyer-Kimling, Rainer, and Kallmann (1966) showed how schizophrenics in New York State followed the general population trend to higher proportions ever married, by comparing a 1934–6 admission sample with one from 1954–6 admissions.

However, the basic reduction in probability of marriage of schizophrenic women before admission remains and the present survey demonstrated more clearly than previous studies that the main factors associated with this reduction were:

1. A schizoid nature which made the normal pattern of heterosexual contacts difficult (as suggested by Ødegaard, 1953, 1960; and by El-Islam and El-Deeb, 1968).
2. A long period between onset of symptoms and hospital admission, during which the patient was obviously unsuitable and unattractive as a marriage partner.
3. Early age at admission, at a time when probability of marriage is high in the general population, thus cutting short the length of the period before admission.

It is surprising that Essen-Möller (1935) found no relationship between age on admission and probability of marriage before illness; schizophrenic women first admitted late in the childbearing period appeared to have a low probability of marriage when they were young, comparable to that of schizophrenic women admitted at an early age. Essen-Möller considered that these results supported Kretschmer's view that very long-standing pre-morbid personality problems occurred in schizophrenics. The present study has clearly demonstrated that the role of such abnormal traits was important in reducing the chance of marriage before admission in some schizophrenics, but that there was a group of schizophrenics of a more normal temperament whose chance of marriage was nearer to that of normal women.

The low probability of marriage among schizophrenic women did not appear to be related to lack of interest in the opposite sex, and the results agree with Popenoe (1928a) in this respect: half of the single schizophrenics who gave adequate information on sexual interest had had at least one serious involvement with a man, and illegitimate fertility was high in this particular sub-group [see CHAPTER XV]. Only one third of the single schizophrenic women had had no such serious relationship, and this was an insufficient proportion to support Mott's (1919) assumption of sexual immaturity in schizophrenics.

The lack of significant differentials between women suffering from affective disorders and the general population in probability of marriage before admission appeared to agree with the similar findings of Essen-Möller (1935) and Ødegaard (1960). A small number of our women suffering from affective disorders, who appeared to be of schizoid temperament, were also less likely to marry than those of a more normal disposition, and although this differential was not of the major importance of that for the schizophrenics, the basic role of personality factors in reducing chance of marriage should be emphasized.

PROBABILITY OF MARRIAGE AFTER ADMISSION

The results on probability of marriage after first admission were also very much as expected on the basis of previous studies, although there was considerable evidence for recent lessening of differentials between patients and normal women. Our schizophrenic women were only 36 per cent as likely to marry as corresponding normal women during this period, which tended to agree with Kallmann's reduced proportions ever married among non-paranoid schizophrenics at the end of his follow-up in Berlin (Kallmann, 1938). Essen-Möller (1935) found a greater difference between his patients in southern Germany and the corresponding general population: his schizophrenic women had a reduced probability of marriage after admission to between one-third and one-ninth of normal. The lessening of differentials found in the present study is no doubt the result of community-orientated psychiatry; and this has been noted by Erlenmeyer-Kimling, Rainer, and Kallmann (1966) in their comparison of pre- and post-war samples in New York State. Unfortunately, they gave no separate analysis of marriage after admission and only showed in a cumulative index that the proportion of ever married schizophrenics was higher in the post-war cohort compared with the pre-war cohort at the end of their follow-up, and that marriage became more frequent among patients as marriage rates increased in the general population.

The present inquiry clearly demonstrated that the crucial factors in reducing the probability of marriage of schizophrenic women after admission were the course of psychosis and personality. First, in respect of course of psychosis, schizophrenic women admitted only once were 74 per cent as likely to marry as normal women compared with the significantly lower probability of 27·8 per cent for those patients admitted between two and none times; schizophrenic women whose hospital stay was short were 53·6 per cent as likely to marry as normal women compared with the more significantly reduced chance of marriage of 16 per cent of normal for long-stay patients. These findings agreed with Essen-Möller's (1935) reduction in chance of marriage to a third of normal for recovered schizophrenics and a ninth of normal or less for deteriorated institutionalized patients. Although even our long-stay cases did not reach such low probabilities, no doubt because they are not so completely deteriorated as those in his follow-up sample, which was seriously biassed towards hospitalized patients.

It is interesting that Essen-Möller (1935) showed that the reduction in probability of marriage after admission was to some extent independent of the effect of hospitalization, although he did not appear to give any definite explanation of this. The above results have also indicated that the reduction in probability of marriage after admission was not solely dependent upon the effect of hospitalization.

The present study clearly demonstrated the role of personality factors in reducing chance of marriage after admission: schizophrenics of markedly introverted nature were only 18·4 per cent as likely to marry as normal women of corresponding age during the same calendar period, whereas those prone to variable moods had a higher chance of marriage (35·6 per cent of normal), and those schizophrenics of more normal temperament were even more likely to marry (56·4 per cent of the normal probability). There appeared to be some slight interaction between normal personality and better prognosis. No previous inquiry has clearly shown the importance of personality in reducing probability of marriage after admission, although Böök (1953) in his study of a north Swedish isolate suggested this indirectly when he explained the higher proportion of married schizophrenic women than expected on the basis of the general population, by the fact that ability to survive the Arctic winters was more important in marriage selection there than more pleasant psychological characteristics such as emotional warmth which the schizophrenic often lacks. The results of the present study would tend to agree with those of El-Islam and El-Deeb (1968), who also recently demonstrated the role of schizoid personality in reducing chance of marriage among a sample of schizophrenics attending an outpatient clinic in Cairo. They gave further support for the role of personality in a study of the method of marriage of male schizophrenics, who had a significant reduction of love marriages compared with arranged marriages in this Arab community. Although their study was based on a small sample and did not separately analyse probability of marriage before and after illness, the authors noted that the pre-morbid schizoid personality was magnified after the onset of the disease, thus seriously limiting the depth and stability of emotional relationships of schizophrenics.

The probability of marriage after admission of women suffering from affective disorders did not differ significantly from that of the general population of corresponding age during the same calendar periods, unlike Essen-Möller's (1935) manic-depressives whose chance of marriage was reduced to half of normal. His sample contained mainly unrecovered cases whereas many of our women with affective disorders were reactive depressives, who were never psychotic and some of whom recovered after one period of treatment. This clinical difference probably partly accounts for the lack of agreement between the present results and Essen-Möller's. The lack of any significant differential between women suffering from affective disorders and normal women in the present study agreed with Stenstedt's (1952) small follow-up survey in a Scandinavian area, in which he found no significant differences in proportions married between manic-depressives and normal women, when variations in age structure were controlled.

It is necessary, in order to analyse probability of marriage after admission in a controlled manner, to have a fairly large sample. However, it was difficult to detect differentials in the case of single women with affective disorders, because patients in this clinical group are generally admitted to hospital when they are middle aged and, like normal women at that age, the single women in this group are unlikely to marry later. In view of the effect of new drugs (antidepressants, tranquillizing drugs, etc.) on the treatment of affective disorders, a significant difference in probability of marriage is unlikely between this group and normal women, although a sub-group of single patients suffering from recurrent psychotic depressions or from recurrent manic-depressive conditions might exhibit some such reduction after admission.

LEGITIMATE FERTILITY BEFORE ADMISSION

The results on fertility were not of the major clinical and social importance as those on marriage. The reduction in fertility of schizophrenics before admission did not appear to be large enough to be socially important: schizophrenics had a mean family size of $1·36 \pm 0·07$ compared with $1·54$ expected in the corresponding general population, controlled for age at and duration of marriage. However, this difference was statistically significant and is in the expected direction when comparisons are made with Kallmann's (1938) cruder estimates of reduced family size of non-paranoid schizophrenics in Berlin. Both Kallmann (1938) and Essen-Möller (1935) analysed the fertility of patients before the widespread use of birth control had produced the decline of the German birth rate, and the differences they obtained between schizophrenics and normal women were greater than those obtained in recent studies. Essen-Möller found the fertility of schizophrenic women before admission to be about half of normal before the fall of the German birth rate; after the spread of birth control he considered there would be a lessening of this differential, as indicated by our results, in agreement with those of MacSorley (1964) on a small English sample and those of Goldfarb and Erlenmeyer-Kimling (1962) and Erlenmeyer-Kimling, Rainer, and Kallmann (1966) in America.

The results of the present inquiry did not support those of Böök (1953), who found a comparatively high legitimate fertility of schizophrenic women in a north Swedish isolate; no birth control was practised there owing to the prevalence of an orthodox puritanical faith, and the area was too atypical to allow any generalizations. Ødegaard (1960) also found a comparatively high fertility before admission of schizophrenics admitted to Norwegian mental hospitals between 1946–55, although he did suggest that this could be due to some bias towards the lower social classes. However, the present inquiry found that all social classes of schizophrenics had a reduced fertility.

Our special analysis emphasized the importance of controlling the relevant variables known to influence fertility in the general population: religion appeared to be of major importance—the Protestant schizophrenics exhibited a significant reduction before admission whereas the Roman Catholic patients with this diagnosis had an increased fertility, although this was not significantly different from that of the normal women controlled for age at marriage and duration of marriage. Previous inquiries have often failed to give such controlled estimates by religion.

The women suffering from affective disorders had no such significant reduction in legitimate fertility before admission and this agreed with the findings of Essen-Möller (1935) on manic-depressives. He considered the lack of a significant differential in this clinical group was because of the later onset of affective psychoses compared with the schizophrenics. It is surprising that Ødegaard (1960) found the legitimate fertility of manic-depressives to be lower than that of schizophrenics before admission and we could find no evidence for this, although controlled comparisons between clinical groups were not considered to be methodologically possible in this study. Ødegaard's sample of women with affective illnesses may have contained fewer patients from the lower social classes whose fertility would be comparatively high. Our women with affective disorders who were married to men in non-manual occupations did have a statistically significant reduction in fertility when compared with the general population, which would accord a little more with Ødegaard's findings. However, it would appear that the fertility before admission of both main clinical groups did not differ to any meaningful sociological extent from that of the corresponding general population.

LEGITIMATE FERTILITY AFTER FIRST ADMISSION

The special analysis of fertility after admission produced results in the expected direction: among the majority of schizophrenics who married before admission there was a statistically significant reduction in fertility. They had a mean family size of 0.37 ± 0.05 compared with 0.52 expected in normal women of corresponding age at marriage and duration of marriage. However, this difference was largely dependent on the effect of hospitalization in reducing exposure to conception. The smaller group of schizophrenic women who married after admission showed no such statistically significant reduction in their fertility. Essen-Möller (1935) also found that the fertility of marriages contracted before admission was reduced after admission, in his sample the reduction was given as 70 per cent of the previous level of fertility. He also found the reduction largely dependent upon hospitalization, although his sample was more biassed towards re-admitted patients than ours, and he could give no estimates for recovered cases. Our study indicated that recovered patients did not have such a reduced fertility as deteriorated patients but there was some evidence that a reduction in fertility after admission occurred quite independently of hospitalization in some groups, for example short-stay patients, as Essen-Möller suggested but was unable to clearly demonstrate. Essen-Möller also found no such significant reduction in the fertility of schizophrenic patients who married after admission, as our study confirmed; these patients were probably those with a better prognosis, whose life is little influenced by their previous illness.

Although these statistically significant differentials were obtained for the schizophrenics, they were not large enough to be sociologically important: there has been a lessening of differences during the period after admission since Essen-Möller's survey (1935) and our survey confirmed the findings of Erlenmeyer-Kimling, Rainer, and Kallmann (1966) that post-war samples of schizophrenics appear to attain a level of fertility never reached by pre-war cohorts, even though the follow-up period for the latter is longer than that for the former. Within the schizophrenics (as found for the period before admission) our Protestant patients had a more reduced fertility than Roman Catholics, and those married to men in non-manual occupations appeared to have a more reduced fertility than that of those married to manual workers when comparisons are made with normal women. Such a reduced fertility among women married to non-manual workers was independent of the effect of hospitalization whereas the reduction found for schizophrenics married to manual workers depended on this factor.

The fact that the present results have demonstrated that the fertility of schizophrenics is significantly below that of the corresponding general population should be emphasized. Research such as that of Shearer et al. (1968), indicating a 366 per cent rise in the fertility rate of women in Michigan mental hospitals, when comparisons are made between 1935-9 and 1960-4 samples should be cautiously assessed. In particular these writers have not emphasized adequately the total reduction in the fertility of schizophrenics in terms of reduced probability of marriage, and total reproductive histories. They claim that 63·6 per cent of the rise in births were from schizophrenic women, but they gave no details of the amount of information on the earlier cohorts compared with the recent ones, the latter samples involved follow-up inquiries which could in themselves increase the chance of re-admission of pregnant schizophrenics. The results of the present survey demonstrate clearly that the total fertility of schizophrenics remained well below that of the corresponding general population during recent years of community-orientated psychiatry in England.

No significant differentials were obtained between the fertility of women suffering from affective disorders after admission and that of corresponding normal women, and our results confirmed those of Essen-Möller in this respect. However, there were differences among the women suffering from affective disorders, as discussed above for the schizophrenics: in particular a small atypical group of long-stay patients with affective illnesses had a reduction in fertility which was very significant statistically, although sociologically this group was too small to be important. Women in this clinical group whose husbands were in non-manual occupations also had a reduced fertility independent of hospitalization during the period after admission.

However, in spite of these variations within our clinical groups, it would appear that any definite reduction in the legitimate fertility of women suffering from affective disorders was too slight to be of sociological or eugenic importance.

SEPARATION AND DIVORCE

The analysis of legitimate fertility was controlled for duration of marriage so that when patients parted from their husbands the duration of this time was compared with marriages of corresponding duration in the general population. The finding that schizophrenics appeared to part from their husbands more frequently than normal women, both before and after admission, suggested that marital disruption was another factor in reducing the total fertility of schizophrenics. Women suffering from affective disorders also demonstrated a higher frequency of divorce and separation before admission than would be expected on the basis of Rowntree's (1964) study of women in the general population, and this may be a factor in reducing the total reproduction of some women in this clinical group.

The results on the schizophrenics agree with Ødegaard's (1953) on admissions to Norwegian mental hospitals in which he found a high frequency of divorced patients among paranoid cases. He analysed case histories mainly covering the period before admission and found some evidence of a causal relationship between pre-morbid symptoms and the illness itself and marital breakdown. In our sample there also appeared to be some relationship between abnormal personalities and proportions parting before first admission; but unlike Ødegaard (1953) during the period after admission there was little evidence for the illness directly causing the separation. Our results on marital disruption of schizophrenics agree with those of Brown et al. (1966) in a recent English survey. As they suggest, the total proportion of schizophrenics who part may be three times that of normal women of corresponding marriage duration.

The increased marital disruption of women suffering from affective disorders was not emphasized so much by Ødegaard (1953) and he did not find the causal relationship between affective disorders and marital breakdown that he obtained for his paranoid patients. The role of personality factors in marital disruption before admission was also not so clear among our women in this clinical group as among the schizophrenics. However, our survey obtained definite evidence for an increased frequency of separation and divorce among women with affective disorders before admission, to the same extent as that found for the schizophrenics, although after admission the former group did not appear to exhibit such important differences.

ILLEGITIMATE FERTILITY

The data on illegitimate fertility appeared to be very much as expected on the basis of Ødegaard's results (1960). Most illegitimate births to schizophrenics were during the period before admission. When illegitimate births were measured as the percentage of total live births to patients the schizo-phrenics appeared to have three times as many illegitimate children as the estimate for women in the general population [see CHAPTER XV]. These births were mainly to schizophrenics who did not have pronounced schizoid person-alities and who appeared to have normal involvements with the opposite sex.

As Ødegaard found, the illegitimate fertility of women with affective dis-orders did not appear as high as that of schizophrenics but this may be solely because more of them had married and thus fewer were exposed to the risk of an illegitimate pregnancy. Unfortunately Ødegaard only gave data on births to single patients whereas this study, and also Essen-Möller's (1935) inquiry, studied illegitimate fertility to married women as well. However, our results did not agree with Essen-Möller's, who found that illegitimate births to patients declined with the general population decline in the birth rate, and after admission there was a greater reduction among schizophrenics than manic-depressives; our women suffering from affective disorders had fewer illegitimate births after admission than the schizophrenics, probably because they were an older group.

The study of illegitimate fertility really required a more detailed analysis than was possible in this survey before any really reliable estimates could be made. There has been a considerable amount of literature suggesting the application of psycho-analytic theory to the assessment of the personality structure of unmarried mothers (Young, 1954). Freud's *Collected Papers* II, p. 191, were quoted by Young as suggesting that the relationship of the unmarried mother to the father of the child was masochistic and a regression to the pre-oedipal situation. The unmarried mother perhaps felt an inferior woman and returned to the anal-sadistic phase, on which beating by the father was a form of sexual gratification. Young did not, however, go into the details of the few *psychotic* girls in his sample of 350 girls and 1,000 case histories. It was very much regretted that there was not time during the present study to undertake an intensive inquiry into the sub-group of our sample having illegitimate children. The role of the broken home was by no means clear, although about a third of our patients had experienced traumatic situations during childhood or adolescence. Vincent (1961) demonstrated that there were as many broken homes among never-pregnant high-school girls and his group of unmarried mothers. It is impossible to review the considerable literature here but Greenland (1957) in a Scottish survey suggested that unmarried mothers were not significantly different from other women of the same age and social class, although they may be perhaps more fecund; they may use contraceptives less carefully or not at all, as Kravitz, Trossmann and Feldmann (1966) had suggested. It is therefore impossible to conclude about the seemingly high illegitimate fertility of the schizophrenic sample, except that the fact that such a large proportion do not marry is the most obvious reason for high illegitimacy.

MMF

GENERAL ASSESSMENT OF RESULTS

In general, the results of the present inquiry tended to confirm those of previous studies in emphasizing definite differential probability of marriage and fertility of schizophrenics, whereas women suffering from affective disorders did not appear to differ significantly from the general population in this respect. The reduced probability of marriage of schizophrenics before admission appeared to be due to the influence of pre-morbid schizoid traits making normal contacts difficult rather than to definite lack of interest in the opposite sex. After admission, the reduction of probability of marriage of the schizophrenics to one-third of that of normal women confirmed the earlier results of Essen-Möller (1935), although the development of community care has considerably lessened the differential between patients and normals. The development of a chronic psychosis significantly reduced the chance of marriage but as Essen-Möller suggested, there appeared a reduction independent of the effect of hospitalization which was probably due to the crucial role of personality in marriage selection. There was a definite statistical reduction in the legitimate fertility of schizophrenics both before and after admission, but this was too slight to be of sociological importance, and these results confirmed those of Erlenmeyer-Kimling, Rainer, and Kallmann (1966) in America emphasizing the impact of community care on lessening differential fertility. Essen-Möller (1935) also suggested the role of birth control in lessening such differentials.

The increased frequency of separation and divorce among schizophrenic women, both before and after their admission, is also a factor in reducing the total fertility of schizophrenics. However, there was considerable evidence that high illegitimate fertility among this clinical group could compensate partially for this.

Women suffering from affective disorders were found to be very similar to women in the corresponding general population in probability of marriage and fertility, both before and after their first admission. However, the importance of analysis by the relevant sociological variables was also demonstrated in this group in that women married to men in non-manual occupations had a reduced fertility, which was statistically significant, and no such reduction was found for women suffering from affective disorders who were married to men in manual occupations. It should be emphasized that there was an increased frequency of separation and divorce among women with these disorders before their first admission, which has not been emphasized by previous studies. The illegitimate fertility of women with affective disorders did not appear to be significantly higher than that expected on the basis of the general population, which confirmed Ødegaard's (1960) results.

CHAPTER XIX

CONCLUSIONS

THIS survey was the first in England to estimate probability of marriage and fertility of women suffering from schizophrenia and affective disorders by the use of reliable mathematical techniques. It was also one of the first surveys in Western societies since the impact of community-orientated psychiatry to assess the total fertility of these clinical groups, involving a separate analysis of trends before and after first admission. The results clearly demonstrated that schizophrenic women were very different from normal women in probability of marriage and fertility, whereas as a whole women suffering from affective disorders did not differ significantly from the general population in this respect.

The basic difference between schizophrenics and normal women was their considerable reduction in probability of marriage to three-quarters of normal before illness and to one-third of normal afterwards. There was variation within the schizophrenic group; those of schizoid personality were less likely to marry before and after illness than those of a more normal temperament; after illness those whose psychosis was chronic were significantly less likely to marry than those who required only one admission. These basic differentials will remain however much community care is developed, because many schizophrenic women are psychologically different from normal women long before the onset of a manifest psychosis, and whether they take their medication or not, the crucial role of personality in marriage selection will always diminish their chance of marriage to some extent.

There was a definite reduction in the legitimate fertility of the schizophrenic women but this was too slight both before and after illness to be of sociological importance. With the spread of birth control and the impact of community care there has been a lessening of fertility differentials between schizophrenics and women in the general population and these patients appear to be replacing themselves more in comparison with the general population than in the days when long-term institutional care characterized the lives of schizophrenics. However, the total fertility of schizophrenics is reduced by a higher frequency of separation and divorce than is found for normal women, but the effect of this reduction may be partially eliminated by the apparently high illegitimate fertility of schizophrenics.

The writer would like to emphasize that the results of this survey indicate that the total reproductive fitness of schizophrenic women, as was measured by probability of marriage and fertility, was still significantly lower than that of corresponding women in the general population. There remains, therefore,

170 DISCUSSION AND CONCLUSIONS

an academic need to depart from monogenic theories of the genetic basis of schizophrenia, and Gottesmann and Shield's (1967) polygenic theory appears at present to be a better model for explaining continuing high incidence of schizophrenia in the light of the evidence in this book of reduced total fertility, because this polygenic theory allows the possibility of mutation rates at different loci within Haldane's estimates of human gene mutability. Moreover, Gottesmann and Shields state that their theory need not involve the search for physiological advantages among schizophrenics, which is at present difficult according to Kuttner and Lorincz (1966) in their note on schizophrenia and evolution. A multi-disciplinary approach involving several genes and considerable environmental precipitants appears the most sensible at the present stage of our knowledge of this problem.

The women suffering from affective disorders were much more similar to normal women, and any differentials which once existed appear now to be minimized. However, women in this clinical group who were of schizoid temperament also appeared less likely to marry before admission than those of a more normal disposition, but the former were a small atypical group. The legitimate fertility of women with affective disorders appeared to be very similar to that of the corresponding general population. However, like the schizophrenic women, this group appeared to be especially prone to marital breakdown *before* illness. The frequency of illegitimate births among the women with the affective disorders did not appear to be greater than that expected on the basis of the general population, although the accuracy of this type of estimate was particularly difficult to assess.

In conclusion, the total reproductive fitness of women suffering from affective illnesses as measured by probability of marriage and fertility appeared to be almost as high as that of corresponding women in the general population, and any differentials which have been found within this clinical group were too small to be of any real sociological or eugenic importance.

REFERENCES

ALLAND, A. (1967) A further note on evolution and schizophrenia, *Eugen. Quart.*, **14**, 2, 158.

ARMSTRONG, C. W. (1927) *The Survival of the Unfittest*, London.

BAILLARGER, M. (1849) On Statistics Applied to the Study of Mental Diseases. Letter to M. Renaudin, Physician and Director of the Asylum for the Insane at Fains (trans. by an inmate of N.Y. State Lunatic Asylum), *Amer. J. Insan.* **5**, 4, 322.

BEAN, L. L. (1966) The fertility of former mental patients, *Eugen. Quart.*, **13**, 1, 34.

BLEULER, E. (1911) *Dementia Praecox, or the Group of Schizophrenias*, trans. Zinkin, J., and Lewis, D. C. (1950) pp. 9-12, 245-55, 269, New York.

BÖÖK, J. A. (1953) A genetic and neuropsychiatric investigation of a N. Swedish population with special reference to schizophrenia and mental deficiency, *Acta Genet. (Basel)*, **4**, 1-139, 345-414.

BOWLBY, J. (1949) *Personality and Mental Illness—an Essay in Psychiatric Diagnosis*, Chapter IV and Appendix A, London.

BROWN, G. W. (1967) The family of the schizophrenic patient, in *Recent Developments in Schizophrenia*, ed. Coppen, A. J., and Walk A., *Brit. J. Psychiat.*, Special Publications No. 1.

BROWN, G. W., BONE M., DALISON, B., and WING, J. K. (1966) *Schizophrenia and Social Care*, Maudsley Monographs, No. 17, Chap. I and VI, London.

BRUGGER, C. (1931) Versuch einer Geisteskrankenzählung in Thürin gen, *Z. ges. Neurol. Psychiat.*, **133**, 351 (as referred to by Essen-Möller, E., 1935).

BURCH, P. R. J. (1964) Schizophrenia, some new aetiological considerations, *Brit. J. Psychiat.*, **110**, 818-24.

CHAPMAN, T. A. (1880) The comparative mortality of different classes of patients in asylums, *J. ment. Sci.*, **113** (New Series 77), 11.

DAHLBERG, C. (1933) Die Fruchtbarkeit der Geisteskranken, *Z. ges. Neurol. Psychiat.*, **144**, 427 (as referred to by Lewis, A. J., 1958).

DARWIN, L. (1926) *The Need for Eugenic Reform*, Chapter XIV, London.

DAYTON, N. (1940) *New Facts on Mental Disorder*, Chapters 6, 7, and Appendix, Baltimore.

EDGEWORTH, E. Y. (1914) Discussion of the paper by Greenwood, N., and Yule, G., *J. roy. statist. Soc.*, **77**, 198.

EL-ISLAM, M., FAKHR, and EL-DEEB, HEND A. (1968) Marriage and fertility of psychotics: a study at an Arab psychiatric clinic, *Social Psychiat.*, 3, 1, 24-7.

ERLENMEYER-KIMLING, L., and PARADOWSKI, W. (1966) Selection and schizophrenia, *Amer. Naturalist*, 100, 916, 651-65.

ERLENMEYER-KIMLING, L., RAINER, J. D., and KALLMANN, F. J. (1966) Current reproductive trends in schizophrenia, in *Psychopathology of Schizophrenia*, ed. Hoch, P. D., and Zubin, J., New York.

ESSEN-MÖLLER, E. (1935) Untersuchungen über die Fruchtbarkeit gewisser Gruppen von Geisteskranken (schizophrenen, manischdepressiven und epileptikern), *Acta psychiat. neurol (Kbh.)*, Supp. VIII, Chapters 3, 4 and 8.

—— (1959) Mating and fertility patterns in families with schizophrenia, *Eugen. Quart.*, 6, 142-7.

FALCONER, D. S. (1965-6) The inheritance of the liability to certain diseases estimated from the incidence among relatives, *Ann. hum. Genet.*, 29, 51.

FARINA, A. (1960) Patterns of role dominance and conflict in parents of schizophrenic patients, *J. abnorm. soc. Psychol.*, 61, 31.

FARR, W. (1835) *Statistics of English Lunatic Asylums and the Reform of their Public Management*, London.

FONSECA, A. F. DA (1959) *Análise Heredo-clinica das Perturbaçoes Afectiva Atraves de 60 Pares de Gémeos*, Faculdade de Medicina, Oporto (as referred to by Shields, J., 1968).

—— (1963) Affective equivalents, *Brit. J. Psychiat.*, 109, 464.

FRANK, C. H. (1965) The role of the family in the development of psychopathology, *Psychol. Bull.*, 64, 191.

FREMMING, K. H. (1951) *The Expectation of Mental Infirmity in a Sample of the Danish Population*, London, (Occasional papers in Eugenics, No. 7).

GARRONE, G. (1962) Étude statistique et génétique de la schizophrénie à Genève de 1910 à 1950, *J. Génét. hum.*, 11, 89.

GENERAL REGISTER OFFICE (1959) *Census, 1951, Fertility Report*. Tables Section C, Married Women aged 45-9 at the Census, Table C, p. 178, London, H.M.S.O.

—— (1960) *Classification of Occupations 1960*, London, H.M.S.O.

—— (1961a) *The Registrar General's Statistical Review for England and Wales for the Two Years 1957-8, Supplement on Mental Health*, Table M10A, p. 12, London, H.M.S.O.

—— (1961b) *Census, 1961, County Report, London*, London, H.M.S.O.

—— (1962) *The Registrar General's Statistical Review of England and Wales for the Year 1959, Supplement on Mental Health*, Appendix Table M24 (i), p. 78, London, H.M.S.O.

—— (1963a) *Census, 1961, County Report, Middlesex*, London, H.M.S.O.

—— (1963b) *The Registrar General's Statistical Review of England and Wales for the Year 1961*, Part II, Tables Population, Table C, p. 10, London, H.M.S.O.

—— (1964) *The Registrar General's Statistical Review of England and Wales for the year 1961 Part III Commentary, Table CXXVIII*, p. 254, London, H.M.S.O.

—— (1965a) *Census, 1961, England and Wales Occupation Industry and Socio-economic Groups for London*, Table 5, London, H.M.S.O.

—— (1965b) *Census, 1961, England and Wales Occupation Industry and Socio-economic Groups for Middlesex*, Table 5, London, H.M.S.O.

GIBBS, C. E. (1924–5) Sexual behaviour and secondary hair in female patients with manic depressive psychoses and the relation of these factors to dementia praecox. *Amer. J. Psychiat.*, **4**, Old series Vol. 81, 41.

GLASS, D. V. Unpublished data from a study of London.

GOLDFARB, M. D., and ERLENMEYER-KIMLING, L. (1962) Mating and fertility trends in schizophrenia, in *Expanding Goals of Genetics in Psychiatry*, ed. Kallmann, F. J., New York.

GOODMAN, N. (1957) Relation between maternal age at parturition and incidence of mental disorder in the offspring, *Brit. J. prev. soc. Med.*, II, 203.

GOTTESMAN, I. I., and SHIELDS, J. (1966) Schizophrenia in twins. 16 years' consecutive admissions to a psychiatric clinic, *Brit. J. Psychiat.*, **112**, 809.

—— (1967) A polygenic theory of schizophrenia, *Proc. nat. Acad. Sci. (Wash.)*, **58**, 1, 199-205.

GRANVILLE-GROSSMAN, K. L. (1966) Parental age and schizophrenia, *Brit. J. Psychiat.*, **112**, 490, 899.

GREENLAND, C. (1957) Unmarried parenthood, *Lancet*, **i**, 148-51.

GREENWOOD, M., and YULE, G. (1914) On the determination of the size of the family; and of the distribution of characters in order of birth from samples taken through members of sibships, *J. roy. statist. Soc.*, 77, 179.

HARRIS, A., NORRIS, V., LINKER, I., and SHEPHERD, M. (1956) Schizophrenia, a prognostic and social study, *Brit. J. prev. soc. Med.*, **10**, 107.

HELGASON, T. (1964) Epidemiology of mental disorder in Iceland, *Acta psychiat. scand.*, Supp. 173, Table 31, p. 85.

HERON, D. (1907) A first study of the statistics of insanity and the inheritance of the insane diathesis, *Eugenics Laboratory, Memoir II*.

HUXLEY, J., MAYR, G., OSMOND, H., and HOFFER, A. (1964) Schizophrenia as genetic morphism, *Nature (Lond.)*, **204**, 220.

KALLMANN, F. J. (1938) *The Genetics of Schizophrenia: a Study of the Heredity and Reproduction of the Families of 1087 Schizophrenics*, Chapters I, II, III, IV and VIII, New York.

KALLMAN F. J. (1946) The genetic theory of schizophrenia; an analysis of 691 schizophrenic twin index families, *Amer. J. Psychiat.*, **103**, 309.

—— (1950) The genetics of psychosis, an analysis of 1,232 twin index cases, *Congrès International de Psychiatrie, Paris 1950, VI Psychiatrie Sociale Génétique et Eugénique*, p. 1, Paris.

KAPLAN, A. R. (1965) On the genetics of schizophrenia, *Eugen. Quart.*, **12**, 3, 132.

KETY, S. S. (1966) Current biochemical research in schizophrenia, in *Psychopathology of Schizophrenia*, ed. Hoch, P. H., and Zubin, J., New York.

KISHIMOTO, K. (1957) A study on the population genetics of schizophrenia, *Proc. 2nd Internat. Congress of Psychiatry*, Vol. 2, Zurich.

KRAVITZ, H., TROSSMANN, B., and FELDMANN, R. B. (1966) Unwed mothers, practical and theoretical considerations, *Canad. psychiat. Ass. J.*, **11**, 6, 456-64.

KRINGLEN, E. (1966) Schizophrenia in twins, an epidemiological-clinical study, *Psychiatry*, **29**, 172.

—— (1968) Twin study in schizophrenia, in *Fourth World Congress of Psychiatry*, Part 2, ed. Lopex Iber, J. J., Internat. Congress Series, No. 150. pp. 1087-90, Excerpta Medica Foundation.

KUTTNER, R. E., and LORINCZ, A. B. (1966) Schizophrenia and evolution, *Eugen. Quart.*, **13**, 4.

LAURENCE, H. M. (1959) Tracing patients, *Lancet*, **ii**, 208.

LEWIS, A. J. (1934) Melancholia. A clinical survey of depressive states, *J. ment. Sci.*, **80**, 278, 258.

—— (1944) Depression, *J. ment. Sci.*, **90**, 256.

—— (1958) Fertility and mental illness (Galton Lecture), *Eugen. Rev.*, **50**, 2, 91.

LIDZ, T., and FLECK, S. (1960) Human integration and the role of the family, in *The Etiology of Schizophrenia*, ed. Jackson, D. D., New York.

LUXENBURGER, H. (1935) Untersuchungen an Schizophrenen Zwillingen und ihren Geschwistern zur Prüfung der Realität von Manifestationsschwankungen, *Z. Neurol.*, **154**, 2 (as referred to by Erlenmeyer-Kimling, L., *et al.*, 1966).

LUYS, J. (1895) Reciprocal morbid attraction of the insane, *Ann. Psychiat.* (as referred to by Meyer, A., 1895).

MACSORLEY, KATE (1964) An investigation into the fertility rates of mentally ill patients, *Ann. hum. Genet.*, **27**, 247.

MALAMUD, W., and RENDER, N. (1939) Course and prognosis in schizophrenia, *Amer. J. Psychiat.*, **95**, 1039.

MAUDSLEY, H. (1862) Genesis of mind, *J. ment. Sci.*, **8**, 61.

MERRELL, D. J. (1951) Inheritance of manic-depressive psychosis, *Arch. Neurol. Psychiat. (Chic.)*, **66**, 272.

MEYER, A. (1895) A review of the signs of degeneration and methods of registration, *Amer. J. Insan.*, **52**, 344.

MOREL, B. A., (1857) *Traité des dégénérescences physiques, intellectuelles et morales de l'espèce humaine*, Paris (as referred to by Lewis, A. J., 1958).

MOTT, F. (1919) Normal and morbid conditions of the testes from birth to old age in one hundred asylum and hospital cases, *Brit. med. J.*, **2**, 698.

MYERSON, A. (1917) Psychiatric family studies, *Amer. J. Psychiat.*, **73**, 3, 355.

NIELSEN, J. (1964) Mental disorders in married couples, *Brit. J. Psychiat.*, **110**, 683

NISSEN, A. J. (1932) Om de schizophrenes fruktbarhetsforhold, *Nord. med.*, **4**, 929 (as referred to by Essen-Möller, E. 1935).

NORRIS, V. (1956) A statistical study of the influence of marriage on the hospital care of the mentally sick, *J. ment. Sci.*, **102**, 147.

ØDEGAARD, O. (1946) Marriage and mental disease, *J. ment. Sci.*, **92**, 35.

—— (1953) New data on marriage and mental disease, *J. ment. Sci.*, **99**, 778.

—— (1960) Marriage rate and fertility in psychotic patients before hospital admission and after discharge, *Int. J. soc. Psychiat.*, **6**, 1 and 2, 25.

PEARSON, K. (1909) *The Scope and Importance to the State of the Science of National Eugenics*, 14th Robert Boyle Lecture (Eugenic Lab. Series I), London.

PENDE, N. (1928) *Constitutional Inadequacies; an Introduction to the Study of Abnormal Constitution*, Chapter 3, p. 74, trans. Naccarati, S., Philadelphia.

PENROSE, L. S. (1956) *Estimate of the Incidence of Cases of Schizophrenia and Manic-depressive Reaction Due to Spontaneous Mutation*, Appendix E, Hazard to Man of Nuclear and Allied Radiations, London, H.M.S.O.

PINEL, P. (1806) *A Treatise on Insanity*, trans. Davis, D. D. (1962), New York.

POPENOE, P. (1928a) Marriage rates of psychotics, *J. nerv. ment. Dis.*, **68**, 17.

—— (1928b) Eugenic sterilization in California; fecundity of the insane, *J. Hered.*, **19**, 73.

RAINER, J. D. (1968) The basic role of genetics in mental health research, *Fourth World Congress of Psychiatry*, Part 2, Lopez Ibor., J. J. Internat. Congress Series, No. 150, pp. 1075-7, Excerpta Medica Foundation.

RENNIE, T. A. C. (1939) Follow-up study of 500 patients with schizophrenia admitted to hospital from 1913-23, *Arch. Neurol. Psychiat. (Chic.)*, **42**, 877.

ROSANOFF, A. M., HANDY, L. M., PLESSET, I. R., and BRUSH, S. (1935) The etiology of so-called schizophrenic psychoses, *Amer. J. Psychiat.*, **91**, 247.

ROSENTHAL, D. (1959) Some factors associated with concordance and discordance with respect to schizophrenia in monozygotic twins, *J. nerv. ment. Dis.*, **129**, 1.

—— (1961) Problems of sampling and diagnosis in major twin studies of schizophrenia, *J. psychiat. Res.*, **1**, 116.

ROSENTHAL, D. (1962) Familial concordance by sex with respect to schizo-
    phrenia, *Psychol. Bull.*, **59**, 5, 401.

ROTHERHAM, D. R. (Ed.) (1962) *Explanatory Manual for the Londoner; a
    Study in Personality and Media*, London.

ROWNTREE, G. (1964) Some aspects of marriage breakdown in Britain during
    the last 30 years, *Pop. Studies*, **18**, 2, 147.

ROWNTREE, G., and CARRIER, N. H. (1958) *The Resort to Divorce in England
    and Wales 1858-1957*, *Pop. Studies*, March, 188.

ROWNTREE, G., and PIERCE, R. M. (1961a) Birth control in Britain. 1. Atti-
    tudes and practices among persons married since the first world war,
    Pop. Studies, **15**, 2, 3.

—— (1961b) Birth control in Britain. 2. Contraceptive methods used by
    couples married in the last 30 years, *Pop. Studies*, **15**, 2, 121.

RUPP, C., and FLETCHER, E. K. (1939-40) A five to ten year follow-up study
    of 641 schizophrenic cases, *Amer. J. Psychiat.*, **96**, 877.

RUTTER, M., and BROWN, G. W. (1966) The reliability and validity of
    measures of family life and relationships in families containing a
    psychiatric patient, *Soc. Psychiat.*, **1**, 1, 38.

SAINSBURY, P. (1955) *Suicide in London; an Ecological Study*, p. 66, Table 13,
    Maudsley Monographs, No. 1, London.

SHEARER, M. L., CAIN, A. C., FINCH, S. M., and DAVIDSON, R. T. (1968)
    Unexpected effects of an 'open door' policy on birth rates of women
    in state hospitals, *Amer. J. Orthopsychiat.*, **38**, 3.

SHIELDS, J. (1968) Psychiatric genetics, Chapter 9 in *Studies in Psychiatry*,
    eds. Shepherd, M., and Davies, D. L., London.

SHIELDS, J., GOTTESMAN, I. I., and SLATER, E. (1967) Kallmann's 1946 schizo-
    phrenic twin study in the light of new information, *Acta psychiat.
    scand.*, **43**, 385-96.

SHIELDS, J., and SLATER, E. (1967) Genetic aspects of schizophrenia, *Hosp.
    Med.*, **1**, 579-84.

SLATER, E. (1958) The monogenic theory of schizophrenia, *Acta genet.
    (Basel)*, **8**, 50.

—— (1966) Expectation of abnormality on paternal and maternal sides in a
    computational model, *J. med. Genet.*, **3**, 3, 159-61.

SLATER, E., and SHIELDS, J. (1953) Psychotic and neurotic illnesses in twins,
    Spec. Rep. Ser. med. Res. Coun. (Lond.), No. 278.

SLATER, E., and WOODSIDE, M. (1951) *Patterns of Marriage*, Chapter 10, p.
    165, London.

STENSTEDT, A. (1952) A study in manic-depressive psychoses—clinical,
    social and genetic investigations, *Acta psychiat. scand.*, Supp. 79.

STEVENS, B. C. (1967) Marriage and fertility of women suffering from
    schizophrenia and affective states; Unpublished Ph.D. thesis, Uni-
    versity of London.

SYLVIUS, J. (1556) In Hippocratis et Galeni physiologiae partem anatomicam isagoge a Jacobo Sylvio conscripta et in libros tres distributa. Hac in recenti editione summa in emendando diligentia est adhibita. Venet. ex off. Erasmiana V Valgrisius.

THURNAM, J. (1845) On the relative liability of the two sexes to insanity, *Amer. J. Insan.*, **3**, 235.

TIENARI, P. (1963) Psychiatric illnesses in identical twins *Acta psychiat. scand.*, **39**, Supp. 171.

TSUANG, M. T. (1967) A study of pairs of sibs both hospitalised for mental disorder, *Brit. J. Psychiat.*, **113**, 283-300.

TUKE, D. H. (1880) On the best mode of tabulating recoveries from insanity in asylum reports, *J. ment. Sci.*, **79**, 115, New series 79, 375.

VINCENT, C. E. (1961) *Unmarried Mothers*, New York.

WALTER, R. D. (1956) What became of the degenerate—a brief history of a concept, *J. Hist. Med.*, **11**, 422.

WEINBERG, W. (1910) Die Rassenhygienische Bedeutung der Fruchtbarkeit, *Arch. Rass.-u. Ges. Biol.*, **7**, 684.

—— (1913) Zur Frage der Messung der Fruchtbarkeit, *Arch. Rass.-u. Ges. Biol.*, **10**, 162 (as quoted by Greenwood, M., and Yule, G., 1914).

WICKSELL, S. D. (1931) Nuptiality, fertility, reproductivity, *Skand. Aktuar. T.*, 135 (as quoted by Essen-Möller, E., 1935).

WING, J. K., DENHAM, J., and MONRO, A. B. (1959) Duration of stay in hospital of patients suffering from schizophrenia, *Brit. J. prev. soc. Med.*, **13**, 145 (Table V, p. 147).

YOUNG, L. (1954) *Out of Wedlock; a Study of the Problems of the Unmarried Mother and her Child*, New York.

ZERBIN-RÜDIN, E. (1963) Zur Erbpathologie der Schizophrenien, *Mitt. Max-Planck Ges. H.*, 1-2, Munich, Max Planck Gessellschaft (as referred to by Erlenmeyer-Kimling, L., *et al.*, 1966).

INDEX

Abortions, therapeutic, in relation to fertility, 101, 114–16

Accuracy of information. *See* Reliability, 149–51

Adequacy of information in case records, 34–5, 149–51

Admission to mental hospitals,
in relation to fertility, 7 et seq., 30 et seq., 34 et seq., 44, 68
in relation to marriage, 5 et seq., 30 et seq., 34 et seq., 44, 68, 70, 89–92

Advantage—hypothesis,
physiological advantage in schizophrenics, 25–6
See Polymorphism

Affective disorders,
analysis of fertility of patients with, 5, 8 et seq., 35, 97 et seq., 132 et seq.
analysis of marriage of patients with, 5, 7, 10 et seq., 34–5, 76 et seq., 119 et seq.
and assortative mating, 139–40
definition of, 44
diencephalic disturbance in, 28
follow-up of patients with, 11 et seq., 50 et seq.
genetic theories of, 28–9
maternal age, 143–5
paternal age, 143–4
suicides among patients with, 140–3
twin studies of, 27–8
See Course of illness; Divorce; Genetics; Illegitimate fertility; Manic-depressive psychosis; Separation; Structure of sample

Age at admission, 105
at first illegitimate birth, 132–3
at first marriage, 64
of patients selected, 44, 68
See Analysis of marriage; Structure of sample

Aims of pilot inquiries, 33–5
of the main study, 38 et seq.

American research,
involving follow-up studies, 5 et seq.

on the marriage and fertility of manic-depressives, 5 et seq.
on the marriage and fertility of schizophrenics, 5 et seq., 165
on unmarried mothers, 167

Analysis,
methods of the fertility analysis, 63–4
methods of marriage analysis, 60 et seq.
of all races, 76 et seq., 85 et seq., 97 et seq.
of British white patients only, 76 et seq., 85 et seq., 97 et seq.
of illegitimate births to patients, 132 et seq.
of marital status changes, 119 et seq.
See Probability of marriage; Statistical methods; Variables

Arab patients,
marriage and fertility of, 20

Arranged marriages
of male schizophrenics in Cairo, 20

Assortative mating,
of women with affective disorders, 139–40
of women with schizophrenia, 139–40

Asylums,
American in the late nineteenth century, 2
English in the nineteenth century, 1–2

Atrophy,
testicular in schizophrenics, 8

Bavaria,
Essen-Möller's survey in, 11 et seq.

Berlin,
Kallmann's study on marriage and fertility of schizophrenics in, 10–11

Bias, 67 et seq.
towards Roman Catholic patients, 73, 75
See Representativeness of the sample

Biochemistry of schizophrenia, 29

Birth control
in Britain, 29, 73
in Germany, 14 et seq.
in relation to religion, 73, 98, 163
not used by unmarried mothers, 167

Birth rate,
  fall in the German birth rate, 14 et seq.
  fall in the illegitimate birth rate in Germany, 15
  illegitimate rate in England and Wales, 134
  increase among American in-patients, 18
  See Fertility; Illegitimate fertility
Births,
  registration of in Bavaria, 11
  See Fertility
Bleuler's concept of schizophrenia, 30
Borken,
  Muckerman's study of fertility in, 11
British white patients
  in the main study, 73, 75
Broken homes,
  and unmarried mothers in America, 167
  experienced by patients having illegitimate children, 136-7
Burden of care of mentally ill,
  on relatives, 30-1

Camberwell,
  social class structure of, 69-73
Camberwell Register
  of psychiatric patients, 69
Cards,
  punching of I.B.M. cards, 65
  See Data processing
Case records
  as source of information, 34, 149-51
Catatonic patients,
  fertility of, 11
  genetics of, 23
  marriage of, 10, 69-73
Catchment area of hospital selected, 36
  population of, 43 et seq.
Causes of death
  among female patients of reproductive age, 140, 142-3
Census data,
  use of in main study, 43-5, 69
  use of in other studies, 5-7, 13, 19
Children of patients,
  effects of parents' illness on, 31
  See Fertility; Illegitimate fertility
Chronic institutionalized schizophrenics,
  fertility of, 35-7
Class, social in Greater London, 44-5, 67-73
  See Social class
Clinical structure of main sample, 67 et seq.

Coding,
  of questionnaires, 64-5
  reliability of, 65
Cohabitation
  among Jamaican patients in relation to illegitimate births, 135
Coloured patients, 73, 75
Community care, 30 et seq.
Computer(s),
  use of, 65
  See Data processing
Conception,
  diminished risk of patients whilst in hospital, 63-4, 105 et seq., 164-6, 169-70
Concepts of degeneracy, 2
Concordance rates,
  in twin studies, 22-4
  See Twin studies
Confidence level, 64
  See Statistical methods
Confusion of problems of fact with moral issues, 2
Contraception. See Birth control
Control samples, 8, 9, 11-13, 35
  See General population
Course of illness, 30 et seq., 67, 70
  See Hospital stay
Criticisms of twin studies in schizophrenia, 23-4

Data processing, 64-5
  quality of, 34, 149-51
  time spent collecting, 47, 50
  type of, 47 et seq.
Death of patients,
  cause of, 140, 142-3
Definition
  of fertility, 4
  of patients selected, 44
Degeneracy,
  origin of concept, 2
  theories of, 2
Deliveries within Michigan's mental hospitals, 18
Dementia praecox, 5, 8
  See Schizophrenia
Demography. See Population
Depressive patients, 9, 44
  See Affective disorders; Manic-depressive psychosis; Suicide
Diagnosis,
  accepted in main study, 44, 46
  changes in 149
  reliability of 148-9
Dimeric theory of schizophrenia, 25
  See Genetics

Discharge,
  fertility after, 105 et seq., 164 et seq.
  marriage after, 85 et seq., 161 et seq.
  See Course of illness; Follow-up study
Divorce,
  increased frequency of, 119 et seq.
    among schizophrenics, 31, 119 et seq.,
    166, 169
    among women with affective illnesses,
    119 et seq., 166, 170
  studies of in the general population, 29,
    123 et seq.
Dizygotic twins,
  with affective disorders, 27–8
  with schizophrenia, 22–4
Dominance of one parent,
  significance of, 31
Dominant gene,
  as basis of affective disorders, 28
  as basis of schizophrenia, 25
  See Genetics
Duration of marriage,
  in relation to fertility, 63–4, 97 et seq.,
    105 et seq.
  in relation to separation and divorce,
    123–5

Early discharge policies,
  effects of, 18, 30–2, 164–5
Early psychic trauma among unmarried
  mothers, 136–7, 167
Early statistics,
  discussion of by French psychiatrists,
    1–2
  of mentally ill patients in America, 2
  of mentally ill patients in England, 1–2
Editing of computer data, 65
  See Reliability of information
Educational level reached by patient, 48
  in relation to legitimate fertility, 63,
    101–2, 110–11
  See Fertility
Effects of mental illness among parents on
  children, 31
Electoral registers,
  use of in follow-up, 50
English samples,
  on fertility, 9–10, 43 et seq., 67 et seq.
  on marriage, 9–10, 43 et seq., 67 et seq.,
    123–5
  on mental illness in London, 7, 145
Epileptics, traumatic,
  sample of relatives of, 11, 13
Ethnic structure of sample, 73, 75
Eugenics, 2–4
  eugenic counselling, 10
  eugenic sterilization, 8, 15

Eugenics Laboratory, England, 3–4
  See Sterilization; Genetics
European samples of patients, 6
  German studies on fertility, 10 et seq.
  German studies on marriage, 7, 10 et
    seq.
  See Scandinavian samples
Evolutionary theories,
  and early statistics, 2–3
  and schizophrenia, 22, 25 et seq., 169–
    70
  and theories of degeneracy, 2
  See Genetics
Executive Councils,
  use of in follow-up study, 51
  See National Health Service
Expected mean family size, 48–9, 55,
    63–4, 97 et seq., 105 et seq.
  See Fertility; General population;
    Statistical methods

Falconer's technique for estimating herit-
    ability of liability to schizophrenia,
    26
  See Population genetics
Family size of patients,
  definition of, 4
  measurement of, allowing for the effect
    of hospital stay, 48–9, 105 et seq.
  measurement of, in relation to general
    population, 48–9, 63–4, 97 et seq.
  See Fertility; Statistical methods
Father of patient,
  age at patient's birth, 143–4
  occupation in relation to unmarried
    mothers, 136
Fecundity of male schizophrenics, 8
Fertility of patients,
  after first admission, 6, 10 et seq., 105
    et seq., 164 et seq., 169–70
  and birth control, 14–15, 29, 98–100,
    108–9
  and genetic theories of schizophrenia,
    22, 25–7, 169–70
  and psychiatric drugs, 32
  before first admission, 6, 8 et seq.,
    97 et seq., 163–4, 169–70
  definition of, 4
  in comparison with women in the
    general population, 48–9, 55, 63–4
  interaction of variables in, 64, 103, 116–
    17
  legitimate fertility, 3–4, 6, 8 et seq., 34
    et seq., 97 et seq., 105 et seq., 163 et
    seq.
  post-war studies of (since 1945), 6, 16
    et seq.

Fertility of patients—*cont.*
    pre-war studies of (before 1939), 6, 8 et
        seq.
    sampling problems associated with, 33
        et seq.
    statistical methods of analysis of, 63–4,
        97, 105–6
    See Affective disorders; American
        studies; Genetics; Hospital stay;
        Illegitimate fertility; Interaction of
        variables; Probability of marriage;
        Scandinavian samples; Schizophrenia
Follow-up studies
    of patients with affective disorders, 11
        et seq., 19–20, 30–1, 50–2, 151 et seq.
    of schizophrenics, 10 et seq., 17 et seq.,
        30–1, 50–2, 151 et seq.
Frequency of sexual intercourse in
    relation to legitimate fertility of
    patients, 101–2, 114–15
Freudian theory in relation to unmarried
    mothers, 136–7, 166–7

Galton Eugenics Laboratory, 3–4
Gene frequency of affective disorders, 28
    of schizophrenia, 24 et seq.
General hospitals,
    use of for sampling controls, 9, 20
General population,
    fertility in relation to patients, 48–9,
        63–4
    marriage in relation to patients, 60–3
    use of general population statistics as
        controls, 7, 9, 11, 13, 17, 35, 43–4
    See Marriage; Fertility
General practitioners,
    use of in follow-up study, 50–1
General results on fertility, 98–9, 106–7
    on probability of marriage, 76–7, 85–6
Genetics,
    Kallmann's research, new data on
        twins, 22–4
    link between schizophrenia and affect-
        tive disorders, 28
    mutation rate of schizophrenic genes,
        25 et seq., 170
    of affective disorders, 27–8
    of schizophrenia, 22–7, 28–9
    polymorphism in schizophrenia, 26
    relevance of to present study, 22 et seq.
    twin studies in, 22–4, 27–8
    See Morbid risk in relatives; Polygenic
        theory of schizophrenia; Twin studies
German samples, 6, 7, 10 et seq.
Greenwood–Yule formula, use of, 3–4,
    8
    See Sibships

Haldane's estimates of mutation rates in
    human populations, 25–6, 169–70
Hebephrenic patients,
    fertility of, 11
    marriage of, 10
Heritability of the liability to schizo-
    phrenia,
    use of Falconer's technique, 26
    See Morbid risk in relatives of patients
Heterogeneity of genetic basis of schizo-
    phrenia, 26–8
    of the main sample, 60
Heterosis, genetics, 26
    See Polymorphism
Homes,
    proportion of broken homes among
        unmarried mothers, 136–7, 167
Homosexuality among schizophrenics, 8
Hospital selected for sampling, 43 et seq.
    catchment area of, 36, 43–5
    its effect on social class of patients, 67–
        73
    reasons for selection, 35, 43
    type of, 43, 67–9
Hospital stay,
    effect on fertility of schizophrenics,
        112–13, 114–15, 164–6, 169–70
    effect on fertility of women with
        affective disorders, 112–13, 114–15,
        164–6, 170
    effect on marriage of schizophrenics,
        89, 91–2, 129, 161–3, 169
    effect on marriage of women with
        affective disorders, 89, 91–2, 129,
        161–3, 169–70
    interaction of, with other independent
        variables, 116–17
    method of measuring in relation to
        decreased exposure to risk of con-
        ception, 48–9, 55
Husbands of patients,
    frequency of mental illness among
        them, 139–40

I.B.M. cards, 64–5
    See Data processing; Punching of cards
Iceland,
    genetic studies in, 25
    study of suicide in, 143
Identification,
    sex role in schizophrenia, 23, 167
Illegitimate fertility,
    after admission, 133
    before admission, 132
    of the general population, 134
    of schizophrenics, 133 et seq.

Illegitimate fertility—*cont.*
  of women with affective disorders, 133
    et seq.
  proportion of all fertility of patients
    compared ¦with general population,
    134
  racial factors in, 135
  role of personality in, 135–6
  role of sexual interest in, 134–5
  See Social origin of unmarried mothers
Illness,
  physical, 46, 48, 119, 139–43
  See Affective disorder; Assortative
    mating; Schizophrenia
Immaturity,
  sexual, in schizophrenics, 8
Incidence of psychosis in social classes,
  67–73, 98–101, 108–10
Independent variables, 62–4
  See Variables
Infertility of patients in comparison with
  the general population, 140–1
Inheritance, 22 et seq.
  See Genetics; Falconer's technique
In-patients,
  at time of follow-up, 67, 70
  chronic institutionalized, 35–7
Information,
  quality of, 33 et seq.
  reliability of, 148 et seq.
Insane,
  registration of in the United States, 2
Institutionalization of chronic schizo-
  phrenics, 17–18, 30–1, 35–7, 70, 89,
  91–3, 112–13, 159 et seq.
Interaction of variables,
  in analysis of schizophrenics, 81, 83,
    94–5, 103, 116–17
  in fertility of schizophrenics, 103, 116–
    17
  in probability of marriage, 81, 83, 94–5
  in recovery from illness, 116–17
Intercourse,
  frequency of sexual, 101–2, 114–15
International Statistical Classification of
  Diseases, 34
Irish patients, 73–5, 98–100, 108–9
  See Roman Catholic patients
Iterative methods of solving maximum
  likelihood equations in the analysis of
  marriage, 61

Judicial separation. *See* Separation

Kallmann's twin studies, 22–3
  in the light of new data, 23–4
Kretschmer's concept of pre-morbid

personality, 13
  in schizophrenics, 13, 16, 20

Lack of sexual drive in schizophrenics, 8,
  134–5
Last discharge from hospital chosen, 106
  et seq., 119 et seq.
Leaves from hospital, 49
  correction for in analysis of fertility, 65
Legitimate fertility. *See* Fertility
Length of hospital stay,
  effect on fertility of schizophrenics, 112
    –13
  effect on fertility of women with
    affective disorders, 112–13
  effect on probability of marriage of
    schizophrenics, 89, 91–2
  effect on probability of marriage of
    women with affective disorders, 89,
    91–2
Length of marriage. *See* Duration of
  marriage
Liability of the two sexes to insanity, 1
Liability to inherit schizophrenia, 26
  See Falconer; Heritability
Liability to variable moods, 76, 78–9,
  87–8, 127–8
  See Pre-morbid personality
Likelihood,
  maximum likelihood equation, 61 et seq.
  See Probability of marriage
Logical consistency checks, 65
  See Editing; Computer
London,
  hospital chosen, 67 et seq.
  studies of marriage and fertility of
    patients in, 7, 9
  studies of maternal age in, 143, 145
  See Third London Survey
Long stay patients, 35–7
  See Hospital stay
Love marriages of schizophrenics in an
  Arab community, 20

Manic-depressive psychosis,
  fertility of patients with, 6, 8, 11 et seq.,
    34–5, 97 et seq., 105 et seq., 132 et seq.
  inclusion of these patients in the
    sample, 44–6, 67–9
  marriage of patients with, 6, 7, 11, et seq.,
    34–5, 76 et seq., 85 et seq.
  See Affective disorders; Depressive
    patients
Marital relationship, 48, 101–2, 110–12
Marital status, 5 et seq., 119 et seq.
  in relation to hospital stay, 7, 67, 70,
    119–23, 129

Marital status—*cont.*
  in the main sample, 67 et seq.
  See Divorce; Separation; Unmarried
    mothers
Marital status changes, 119 et seq.
  after admission of schizophrenics, 119
    et seq.
  after admission of women with affective
    disorders, 119 et seq.
  age at first marriage and, 125
  and family size, 127
  before admission of schizophrenics, 119
    et seq.
  before admission of women with
    affective disorders, 119 et seq.
  general population studies of, 123–5
  general results, 119–23
  previous studies of, 7, 16, 20, 30–1
  See Divorce; Probability of marriage;
    Separation; Widowed patients
Marriage,
  after first admission, 85 et seq.
  before first admission, 76 et seq.
  general results on, 76
  methodological problems in studying,
    60–3
  previous studies of, 5 et seq.
  role of personality in selection, 76–9,
    87–8
  See Arranged marriages; Probability of
    marriage
Masculine distribution of pubic hair in
    schizophrenic women, 8
Maternal age,
  of schizophrenic women, 143, 145
  of women with affective disorders, 143,
    145
Maudsley's concept of degeneracy, 2
Maximum likelihood equations,
  in the analysis of probability of
    marriage, 61–2
  See Probability of marriage
Mean age at first illegitimate birth, 132–3
Mean family size, definition of, 4
  See Fertility
Measurement,
  of fertility, taking into account the effect
    of hospital stays, 48–9, 55, 105 et
    seq.
  of onset, 49, 78, 80–1, 89–90
  of personality, 47, 76–9, 87–8, 127–8,
    135–6
  of social class, 48, 98–100, 108–10
  See Methodology; Statistical methods;
    Variables
Mendelian ratios, 24–5
  See Genetics

Mental hospitals, 1, 3, 5 et seq., 29
  and community psychiatry, 30 et seq.,
    159 et seq., 169–70
  in relation to social class of patient,
    67–73
  open door policy, 18
  type of, 35
Mental illness in husband of patient, 139–
    40
  See Affective disorders; Depressive
    patients; Diagnosis; Genetics;
    Manic-depressive psychoses; Rela-
    tives; Schizophrenia
Methodological criteria in the main study,
    33, 43 et seq.
  See Follow-up study
Methodology,
  of the analysis of legitimate fertility,
    63–4
  of the analysis of marital status changes,
    119 et seq.
  of the analysis of probability of
    marriage, 60–3
  of the design of the questionnaire, 47
    et seq.
  of the follow-up study, 50–1
  problems of, 33 et seq., 35, 43 et seq.,
    51–2, 60 et seq.
  See Interaction of variables; Statistical
    methods; Variables
Michigan mental hospitals,
  deliveries to patients in, 18
Ministry of Pensions and National
    Insurance,
  use of in follow-up studies, 51
Model, mathematical
  in the analysis of probability of marri-
    age, 60–3
  See Parameter; Probability of marriage
Monozygotic twins,
  with affective illnesses, 27–8
  with schizophrenia, 22–4
  See Twin studies
Monte Carlo simulation, 61
  See Methodology of marriage analysis;
    Statistical methods
Morbid risk,
  in relatives of patients with affective
    disorders, 28–9
  in relatives of schizophrenics, 24 et seq.
  in the general population, 22, 24, 25–7
  See Weinberg's method of calculating;
    Assortative mating; Falconer's tech-
    nique; Genetics; Population genetics
Mortality,
  cause of in main sample, 140–3
  in relation to fertility, 16, 18

Mortality—*cont.*
  in the nineteenth century, 1–2, 10
  See Cause of death; Suicides
Munich Psychiatric Clinic, 11 et seq.
Mutation rate,
  in humans, 25, 170
  in relation to fertility, 25–7, 170
  of gene for affective disorders, 28
  of schizophrenic gene, 25–7, 170
  See Genetics; Polygenic theory of
    schizophrenia; Population genetics

National Health Service,
  central register, 51
  executive councils, 51
  general practitioners, 50–1, 151 et seq.
  See Follow-up study
New Haven area, United States,
  study of fertility of patients in, 18
New York State,
  ongoing survey of marriage and fertility
    of schizophrenics in, 17–18
  See American studies
Non-response, 151 et seq.
Northern Sweden,
  study of fertility of patients in, 19 et
    seq.
  See Scandinavian samples
Norway,
  studies of marriage and fertility of
    patients in, 16–17
  See Scandinavian samples
Notation used in analysis of marriage,
  61–2
Number of admissions,
  and interaction with other variables,
    94–5
  and probability of marriage, 89, 91
  See Hospital stay

Occupation,
  of patient, 17, 18, 19, 48, 69–73, 98–
    101, 108–10
  of patient's father, 56, 136
  of patient's husband, 48, 69–71, 98–
    101, 108–10, 126–7, 153, 156, 165
  See Social class; Social origins
One-parameter model, 61
  See Probability of marriage; Statistical
    methods
Onset, measurement of, 49

Parameter,
  one-parameter model in the analysis of
    marriage, 61
  two-parameter models in the analysis
    of marriage, 61

  See Statistical methods
Paranoid affective disorders, 44
Paranoid schizophrenics, 69
  fertility of, 11
  marriage of, 10
Paternal age,
  in schizophrenia, 143–4
  in women with affective disorders,
    143–4
Patients,
  physically ill, 46, 119
  See Follow-up; Questionnaire; Psy-
    chiatry; Reliability of information
Periodic psychoses,
  affective disorders, 44, 67–9, 148–9,
    149–51
  depression, 44–6, 67–9
  See Manic-depressive psychoses
Personality,
  and divorce and separation, 127–8
  and reduced probability of marriage,
    76–9, 87–8
  pre-morbid, 47
  See Affective disorders; Illegitimate fer-
    tility; Interaction of variables; Pro-
    bability of marriage; Schizophrenia
Physical illness, 46, 119
Physiological advantage hypothesis
  among schizophrenics, 26
  See Genetics; Polymorphism; Evolu-
    tion
Pilot inquiries, 33 et seq.
Pinel's contribution to early statistics, 1
Polish patients,
  exclusion of in analysis of British
    whites, 73–5
Polygenic theory of schizophrenia, 25–7,
  169–70
Polymorphism,
  genetic in schizophrenia, 26
  See Heterosis; Physiological advantage
    of schizophrenia
Pool, gene, in populations, 25 et seq.
Population,
  calculation of expected fertility in,
    48–9, 55, 63–4, 97–9, 105–7
  calculation of expected probability of
    marriage in, 60–2
  general population statistics as control
    group, 9, 13, 17, 35, 48–9, 63–4
  marital status changes in the general
    population, 29, 123–5
  parameters, 61–2
  samples, 6, 9, 11–13, 67 et seq., 123,
    140, 167
  See Probability of marriage; Statistical
    methods

Population genetics,
  relevance of to main study, 22 et seq.,
    169–70
  review of Falconer's technique, 26
  See Genetics; Mutation rate; Twin
    studies
Post-psychotic period,
  measurement of in fertility analysis,
    63–4, 106 et seq.
  measurement of in marriage analysis, 62
Post-war samples of patients, 5 et seq.
  in comparison with pre-war samples,
    17 et seq.
Postal follow-up study, 50–2, 58
  response rates, 67, 69, 151 et seq.
Pre-psychotic period,
  measurement of in fertility analysis,
    63, 97 et seq.
  measurement of in marriage analysis,
    62, 76 et seq.
Pre-morbid personality, 47
  See Personality
Pre-war sample of patients, 5 et seq.
  difficulties of follow-up, 37
Probability of marriage,
  in relation to total fertility of schizo-
    phrenics, 5 et seq., 169
  interaction of variables in, 81, 83, 94–5
  method of analysis, 60 et seq.
  of schizophrenic women after illness,
    85 et seq.
  of schizophrenic women before illness,
    76 et seq.
  of women with affective disorders after
    illness, 85 et seq.
  of women with affective disorders
    before illness, 76 et seq.
Problems of methodology, 33 et seq., 43
  et seq., 50 et seq., 60 et seq.,
  See Course of illness; Hospital stay;
    Personality; Sampling; Statistical
    methods; Variables
Proportions,
  divorced and separated, 119 et seq.
  ever married, 119–20
  followed-up, 151 et seq.
  See Affective disorders; Schizophrenia;
    Statistical methods
Psychiatric drugs, 30, 32, 159
Psychiatry,
  community orientated, 30 et seq., 159,
    161 et seq.
  development of, 30 et seq.
Psychopathology of unmarried mothers,
    136–7
  See Freudian theory
Psychoses,

affective, 34–5, 44, 46, 67–9
  depressive, 34–5, 44, 46, 67–9
  manic-depressives, 34–5, 44, 46, 67–9
  organic, 33
  periodic, 34–5, 44, 46, 67–9
  schizophrenic, 33 et seq., 44, 46, 67–9
Punching of cards, 65
  See Data processing

Questionnaire, 53–9
  description of, 47 et seq.
  design of in relation to aims, 38, 47 et
    seq.
  design of in relation to data processing,
    64 et seq.
  use in follow-up, 50 et seq.

Race of patients, 73–5
  importance in analysis of illegitimate
    births, 135
  special analysis of British white patients,
    75, 76, 85, 97 et seq., 106 et seq.
Random sampling, 11, 17, 33 et seq., 44,
    67–8, 123, 125
Rates,
  of divorce and separation, 29, 119 et
    seq., 166
  of fertility, 9 et seq., 16–17, 163 et seq.
  of illegitimate births, comparing
    patients and normal women, 9, 15,
    17, 132 et seq., 166–7
  of marriage, 5 et seq., 159 et seq.
  of suicide, 140, 142–3
  See Measurement; Methodology
Ratio of patients' probability of marriage
    to that of normal women, 61 et seq.
  See Analysis; Probability of marriage
Reactive depression, 44–5, 67–9, 125
Recessive gene as basis of schizophrenia,
    24–5
  See Genetics
Recovered patients, 67, 70, 92–5, 114–15,
    151 et seq.
Register,
  of electors, 50
  of National Health Service patients, 51
  of psychiatric patients in Camberwell,
    69 et seq.
  See National Health Service
Registrar General's Statistical Estimates
    for England and Wales, 9, 35, 37, 48–9,
    97–9
Registration,
  of births in Germany before the Second
    World War, 11, 14
  of insane in nineteenth-century,
    America, 2

Registration—*cont.*
  of marriage in Germany before the
    Second World War, 10, 11–13
Relation of fertility
  to genetic theories of schizophrenia, 22
    et seq., 169–70
Relatives of patients, morbid risk in, 22
  et seq.
  response from in follow-up, 151 et seq.
  See Assortative mating; Husbands
Relevant variables,
  in fertility analysis, 63–4
  in illegitimate fertility, 134 et seq.
  in marriage analysis, 60 et seq.
  in separation and divorce, 123 et seq.
  See Variables
Reliability of information, 148 et seq.
Religion of patients,
  and birth control, 29, 98, 100, 108–9
  importance in the analysis of fertility,
    18, 19, 98, 100, 108–9, 163 et seq.
  See Bias; Methodology of fertility
    analysis; Roman Catholics
Representativeness of sample, 67 et seq.
  of follow-up results, 151 et seq.
  See Follow-up study; Non-response
Reproductive rate,
  Ødegaard's method, 16–17
  See Fertility; Total fertility
Response rates, 151 et seq.
Results of present study in relation to
  previous inquiries, 159 et seq.
Role,
  leading to engagement and marriage,
    20, 76–9, 87–8, 159 et seq.
  marital, 101–2, 110–12, 123, 129–30, 166
  of variables in the analysis, 76 et seq.,
    87 et seq., 98 et seq., 108 et seq.,
    123 et seq., 134 et seq.
  parental, 31
  See Probability of marriage; Fertility;
    Variables
Roman Catholic patients, 73–4, 98–100,
  108–9, 125–6, 156, 163–4
  bias towards, 73–5, 156

Sample,
  clinical structure of, 67–9
  marital status and structure of, 67–71
  religious structure of, 73–5
  representativeness of, 67 et seq.
  social structure of, 69
  type of, 44
  See Sibships
Sample size, estimation of, 46
Sampling, frame, 44
  importance of method, 37, 43 et seq.

of general population, 9, 11–13, 18, 19,
  29, 67–73, 123, 167
  pilot studies in, 33 et seq.
Scandinavian samples, 6, 8–9, 16–17, 19–
  20, 143
Schedule, 53–9
  See Questionnaire
Schizophrenia,
  analysis of fertility, 97 et seq., 105 et
    seq., 132 et seq.
  analysis of marriage, 76 et seq., 85 et
    seq.
  and assortative mating, 27, 139–40
  and community care, 30 et seq., 159 et
    seq.
  biochemistry of, 29
  definition of patients selected, 44, 67–70
  genetic theories of, 24 et seq.
  maternal age in, 27, 143–5
  paternal age in, 143–4
  physiological advantage in, 26
  suicides among patients with, 140,
    142–3
  twin studies of, 22 et seq.
  See Course of psychosis; Divorce;
    Illegitimate fertility; Hospital stay;
    Probability of marriage; Separation;
    Structure of sample
Schizophrenia simplex, 10–11
Separation, 119 et seq.
  See Divorce
Sexual drive, 134–5
  lack of in schizophrenic men, 8
Sexual intercourse,
  frequency of in relation to legitimate
    fertility, 101–2, 114–15
Sexual interest, 134–5
  See Unmarried mothers
Sexual needs of women, 29
Sibs,
  of schizophrenics, proportion mentally
    ill, 24, 28–9, 146
  of women with affective disorders,
    proportion mentally ill, 28–9, 146–7
Sibships of patients, 3
  estimation of mean size, 3–4, 8
  See Greenwood–Yule formula
Significance tests, 3–4, 19, 76 et seq., 87
  et seq., 98 et seq., 123 et seq.
  between fertility of patients and women
    in the general population, 64
  See Statistical methods
Single patients. *See* Probability of mar-
  riage
Social change, 29 et seq.
Social class,
  in relation to fertility, 98–100, 108–10

Social class—*cont.*
  measurement of in married patients, 67–72
  measurement of in single patients, 71–3
Social origin of unmarried mothers, 136, 167
Statistical methods,
  in the analysis of fertility, 48–9, 55, 63–4
  in the analysis of probability of marriage, 60 et seq.
  significance tests in, 63–4, 78, 97, 123, 129
  theoretical considerations of, 61–2
Statistics, early, 1 et seq.
Status, marital, 5 et seq., 67–71
  changes in, 119 et seq., 166, 169–70
  See Divorce; Separation
Status, social,
  See Social class; Social origin
Stays in hospital,
  effect on fertility, 47–8, 105 et seq.
  See Hospital stay
Sterility. *See* Infertility
Sterilization and legitimate fertility, 101, 114, 116
Structure of sample, 67 et seq.
  See Sample
Suicide,
  frequency of, by diagnosis, 140, 142–3
Survival of the fittest, 1–2, 170
Sweden,
  fertility of patients, 6, 8–9, 19–20
  studies of marriage, 6, 8–9, 19–20

Testicle atrophy in schizophrenics, 8
Tests, statistical. *See* Statistical methods
Theoretical considerations in the mathematical models of the marriage analysis, 61 et seq.
Therapeutic abortions and sterilizations. *See* Abortions; Sterilizations
Therapy, psychiatric
  in relation to community care, 29 et seq.
  in relation to fertility, 17 et seq., 163 et seq.
Third London Survey, 67 et seq.
Thuringia,
  census of psychiatric patients in, 7
Total fertility,
  components of, 5, 16, 169–70
  See Fertility; Illegitimate fertility; Marital status changes; Probability of marriage
Twin studies, 22 et seq.
  criticisms of, 23–4
  of affective disorders, 27–8
  of schizophrenics, 22 et seq.

relevance of, 22 et seq.
  See Dizygotic twins; Genetics; Monozygotic twins
Two-parameter model, 61–2

Unmarried mothers,
  among patients with affective disorders, 132 et seq.
  among patients with schizophrenia, 132 et seq.
  and early psychic trauma, 136–7, 167
  and racial factors, 135
  and social origins, 136
  See Birth control; Broken homes; Freudian theory; Illegitimate fertility
Urban samples, 6, 7 et seq., 18, 27, 29–30, 33 et seq., 67 et seq., 143

Validity of data, 148 et seq.
  See Reliability of information
Variables, independent,
  age, 5, 7, 13 et seq., 33–4, 38, 47 et seq., 68, 80–1, 87, 89, 97 et seq., 125, 127, 133 et seq.
  course of illness, 10–11, 14 et seq., 30, 40–2, 70, 92–3, 114–15, 153–4, 161 et seq.
  fertility analysis, 48–9, 55, 63–4, 98 et seq., 108 et seq., 132 et seq.
  hospital stay, 15, 17, 18, 30, 39, 67, 70, 89–91, 112 et seq., 129, 161 et seq.
  marriage analysis, 60 et seq., 76 et seq., 87 et seq., 160 et seq., 169 et seq.
  personality, 13–14, 16, 20, 38, 47, 76 et seq., 87–8, 127, 135–6, 151–2, 160–2, 169–70
  religion, 18–19, 40, 73–5, 98–100, 108–9, 125–6, 156, 163–4
  social class, 11, 13, 17, 18, 20, 40, 48, 67 et seq., 98–100, 108–9, 126–7, 153–6, 164 et seq.
  See Relevant variables

Weinberg's method of calculating morbid risks in relatives, 23
Western societies,
  social change in, 29–30
Wicksell's formulae for correction of marriage rates,
  as referred to by Essen-Möller, 14
Widowed patients,
  proportion in each main clinical group, 125

X^2 use of in small samples, 3–4

Young patients, 68
  divorce and separation among, 127, 129